Nursing Is Caring

Nursing Is Caring

Beverly Wheeler, MSN, RN, ACNS-BC

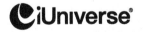

NURSING IS CARING

Copyright © 2015 Beverly Wheeler, MSN, RN, ACNS-BC.

All rights reserved. No part of this book may be used or reproduced by any means, graphic, electronic, or mechanical, including photocopying, recording, taping or by any information storage retrieval system without the written permission of the publisher except in the case of brief quotations embodied in critical articles and reviews.

The views expressed in this work are solely those of the author and do not necessarily reflect the views of the publisher, and the publisher hereby disclaims any responsibility for them.

iUniverse books may be ordered through booksellers or by contacting:

iUniverse
1663 Liberty Drive
Bloomington, IN 47403
www.iuniverse.com
1-800-Authors (1-800-288-4677)

Because of the dynamic nature of the Internet, any web addresses or links contained in this book may have changed since publication and may no longer be valid. The views expressed in this work are solely those of the author and do not necessarily reflect the views of the publisher, and the publisher hereby disclaims any responsibility for them.

Any people depicted in stock imagery provided by Thinkstock are models, and such images are being used for illustrative purposes only.
Certain stock imagery © Thinkstock.

ISBN: 978-1-4917-7524-0 (hc)
ISBN: 978-1-4917-7525-7 (e)

Library of Congress Control Number: 2015913402

Print information available on the last page.

iUniverse rev. date: 11/19/2015

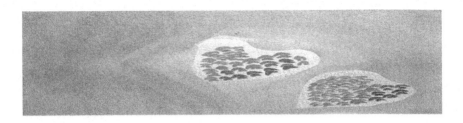

Dedication

This book is dedicated to my late husband, Wylie Thompson. When I first told him my idea for this book, his comment was "Go for it" and then reminded me that I would need patience. He supported me, encouraged me, and frequently reminded me to have patience throughout the major portion of this process. Even though he didn't get to see the finished product, he had read all the students' works and saw the majority of the artist's work. I thank him for his faith in me.

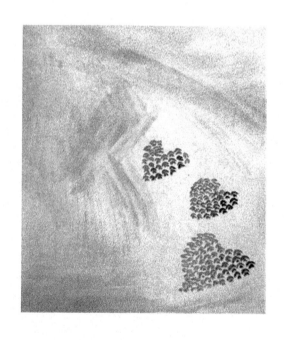

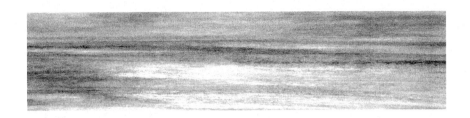

Acknowledgements

I wish to acknowledge and thank Ms Lark Ford, PhD, MSN, MS, RN, a Clinical Assistant Professor at University of Texas Health Science Center at San Antonio, School of Nursing for her suggestion that these students' works be put into a book. Her suggestion started the process. I also want to thank her for her continued enthusiasm, support, and always being ready to give me advice, help, and to answer my questions.

I also want to thank Dr. Carol [Reineck] Huebner, PhD, RN, my Department Chair at the Health Science Center when I started this project, for her excitement and support.

I further want to acknowledge and thank Ms Melissa Maschke, my artist, for the donation of her time and talent in helping me with this project. I wish her the very best as she progresses in her career.

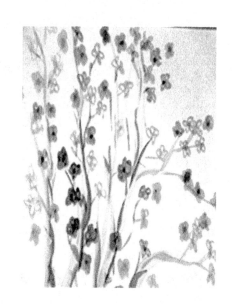
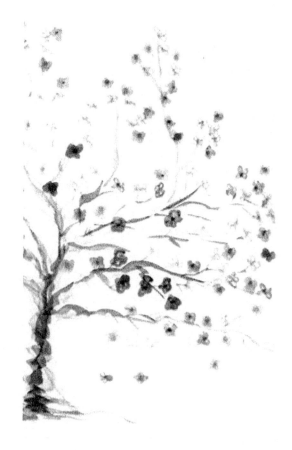

Preface

Most nurses have a patient they will, for a variety of reasons, never forget. When I first started teaching clinical nursing in Virginia, my students and I often talked about patients they would remember and the reasons why they would not forget them.

When I moved to Texas and started teaching, I decided to have all my fourth semester clinical students write a short paper about "**a patient they had taken care of since entering nursing school who had inspired them and made them realize they were in the right profession.**" They also had to give me permission to show their work to others.

When I mentioned to Dr. Carol [Reineck] Huebner, my department chief at that time, what my students were writing, she stated she would like to read them. Each semester after she had read their papers she would pick one of the student's works and print it in the department newsletter. However, as I read their papers I wished more people could read all of the students' papers and see what I was reading. I have cried more than once while reading a very touching paper. After a few semesters, I began to think of possible ways that others could read these papers. Even some of the students stated they wished people knew why we are nurses. Unfortunately, all my ideas had multiple reasons why they would not work.

Finally, one day I was mentioning these papers to Ms. Lark Ford, PhD, MSN, MS, RN, another faculty member, and she immediately stated what a great book of memoirs those papers would make. That suggestion started me thinking and planning. By the next morning I had a plan, and over the next three years this book has become a reality. This book contains the work of the majority of my former students. My goal was to publish one hundred present. Unfortunately, there were some former students whose present addresses I could not find or my letters containing copyright release forms were simply not returned.

I had further difficulty finding an artist who was able to donate his/her time and efforts to help me on this project. The person who volunteered is a student herself.

This book contains the work of nursing students between the Fall 2008 and Spring 2014. Since it is their work and not mine, **100%** of all royalties from this book will go directly to the University of Texas Health Science Center at San Antonio, School of Nursing Scholarship Fund.

Beverly Wheeler, MSN, RN, ACNS-BC
Clinical Assistant Professor, School of Nursing
Department of Health Restoration and
Care Systems Management
University of Texas Health Science Center
San Antonio, Texas

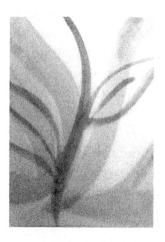

Contents

	Page
Dedication	v
Acknowledgements	vii
Preface	ix

Patient Memories

Anders, Haley. BNS, RN, – A Little Girl's Words	3
Auman, Andrea (Johnson), BSN, RN, – He Was My Very First Patient	4
Ballard, Theresa B, MSN, RN, – My True Calling in Nursing	6
Bermudez, Leonardo, BSN, RN, – A Patient's Poem	7
Cannon, Kristen BSN, RN – A Wonderful Experience	9
Carey, Laura, BSN, RN – A Great Patient	10
Chaiya, Charles BSN, RN, – A Patient I Won't Forget	12
Chavez, Charisa, BSN, RN – Patient Impact in Nursing	13
Cortinas, April BSN, RN, – A Patient To Remember	15
Cunningham, Christina, BSN, RN – An Apology	17
Dearinger, Carla, BSN, RN, – Comeback Kid	18
DeMase, Gillian, BSN, RN, – Miracle of Birth	20
Deuel, Natalie, BSN, RN, – A Most Inspiring Patient	21
Edwards, Yashika Denise, BSN, RN – School Experience	22
Engle, Julie BSN, RN – A Patient's Fears	23

Evans, Tammy, BSN, RN – Confirmation	24
Fulton, Karen B., BSN, RN – Confirmation Of My Chosen Path As An RN	26
Garcia, Jacob BSN, RN – Personal Narrative	28
Garrison, Jessica BSN, RN, – That One Patient	29
Gillespie, Mary Jane, BSN, RN, – Voices of the Voiceless	30
Gorychka, Elizabeth, BSN, RN, – Giving Comfort	32
Greer, Andrea, BSN, RN, – A Patient Remembered	33
Hajda, Sara, BSN, RN – A Man Who Made a Lasting Impression	35
Henk, Krystal (Wohlfahrt), BSN, RN – A Simple Conversation	36
Hines, Kelly, BSN, RN, – My Most Memorable Patient	37
Idicula, Jenny, BSN, RN, – Paralyzed	39
Ingle, Elyse, BSN, RN, – Brief Paragraph	41
Jacob, Feba, BSN, RN – Finding Inspiration	42
Kakuta, Minami, BSN, RN – A Mission Trip	43
Kanarch, Rima, BSN, RN – A Patient's Impact	45
Kirkwood, Chelsea, BSN, RN, – Unconditional Care	46
Kluger, Sharon BSN, RN, – The Moments That Make Life Meaningful	48
Knapp, Katherine, – My First Patient	49
Kruse Jessica Christensen, BSN, RN – Experiences in the Pediatric Intensive Care Unit	50
LaSalle, Nicole, BSN, RN, – A Critically Ill Patient	52
Ledbetter, Lindsey, BSN, RN, – A Patient Who Made A Difference	53
Lee, Eun, BSN, RN, – A touching story	54
Lundy Zeinelabdin, Lucinda, BSN, RN, – I Learned to Listen	55

Manocchio, Antonio, BSN, RN, – A Grateful Patient	57
Martinez, Jesus BSN, RN, – A Special Patient	58
Medintz, Jackie BSN, RN, – A Pediatric Patient	59
Michalec, Karen, BSN, RN, – A Patient Who Inspired Me	60
Micheletti, Tanya, BSN, RN, – My "A Ha Moment"	61
Micke, Luka, MSN, RN, – A Fun and Genuine Patient	62
Moon, Crisann (Dodgen) BSN, RN, – Angels	63
Moreno, Allison BSN, RN, – A Wound Care Patient	64
Neri, Rocio M, BSN, RN, – A Spanish Speaking Patient	65
Ojowa, Winifred BSN, RN, – My Inspiration	66
Olsen, Kristin, BSN, RN, – Inspiring Patient Experience	68
Omisola, Kristina, BSN, RN, – A Young Soldier	69
Paglia, Alaina BSN, RN, – A Little Boy	70
Perez. Krystal, BSN, RN, – Significant Patient	71
Pitts, Kelleah, BSN, RN, – My Labor and Delivery Patient	73
Polasek, Jennifer, BSN, RN, – Answers	74
Powao, Reynaldo BSN, RN, – An Angry Patient	76
Ramos, Analisa, BSN, RN, – Fluff Is Good Medicine	77
Richesin, Alicia, BSN, RN, – A Touching Patient	79
Roberson, Takesha, BSN, RN, – A Little Girl in PICU	80
Robisheaux, Ryan, BSN, RN, – Nursing Experience	82
Sakhel, Emil, BSN, RN, – Patient Who Touched Me As A Student	84
Saldivar, Melodie, BSN, RN, – My Patient Inspired Me	85
Sheesley, Martita, BSN Nursing Student, – My "A HA" Moment	86
Silva, Keyster, BSN, RN (US Army Nurse) – Babies Depend on Nurses	88

Sirchia, Erika, BSN, RN, – The Patient That Changed My World ... 89

Smith, Rodney, BSN, RN, – Patient Who Touched Me as a Student ... 91

Solis, Eli, BSN, RN, – Why Nursing Is For Me ... 92

Stefanic, Meaghan BSN, RN, – One Patient Vividly Remembered ... 93

Stuckey, Kristi, BSN, RN, – A Special Child ... 94

Sylvester, Chris, BSN, RN, – A Patient That Touched Me ... 96

Taele, Josephine, BSN, RN, – My Niche ... 97

Talley, Sara, BSN, RN, – A Little Brother ... 99

Teran, Meghan , BSN, RN – A Patient Who Helped Me Realize I Chose the Right Career ... 100

Theriot, Kimberly, BSN, RN – My Most Memorable Patient ... 101

Thomas, Antony, BSN, RN, – A Memorable Couple ... 102

Thomas, Ashley. BSN, RN, – My First Code Blue ... 103

Turner, Christela, BSN, RN, – Patient Reflection ... 104

Vaello, Kathryn [Lawson], BNS, RN – Unforeseeable Forces ... 105

Valle. Angelica, MSN, RN, – An Uncooperative Patient ... 107

VanBremen, Russell, BSN, RN, – A Homeless Patient ... 108

Villasenor Raquel, BSN, RN – A Busy Day ... 109

Wholly, Amanda, BSN, RN (US Air Force) – Intensive Care Unit Mother ... 111

Zorn, Kristy, BSN, RN, – A Very Bad or Bored Patient ... 112

A Challenge ... 115

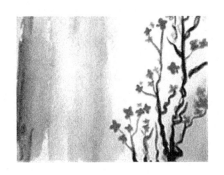

Patient Memories

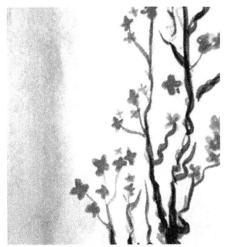

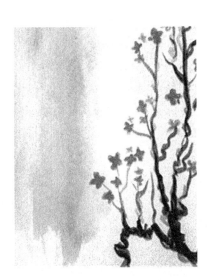

A Little Girl's Words

I distinctly remember the moment that I knew I wanted to become a nurse. It was the summer of 2008, and I was a camp counselor at a special needs camp talking care of a camper for the week. Seeing a young child, who was told would never have a "normal" life due to mental and physical disabilities, sincerely enjoy and live life to the fullest was truly astonishing. I knew in that moment I wanted to live the rest of my life working in an occupation that would allow me to help people achieve their goals not only in health but in life.

A couple of years later, I found myself in nursing school. I knew I was in the right profession but I was confused as to which area I wanted to practice. I originally started out wanting to do labor and delivery, but I quickly realized that I liked everything! My third semester I had my pediatric rotation and was introduced to the patient that changed my life. She was a young girl who refused to be defined by her illness. Despite having several surgeries, illnesses, and pain crisis', she had the most paramount outlook on life. Her happiness and laughter was contagious, and I found myself in her room for the entire duration of my shift. She told me stories about her life going beyond her illness, and I helped her beyond just the pain and actually listened to her in which I don't think a nurse ever had. By the end of my shift she told my teacher that she knew I was going to be a great nurse and that she couldn't wait to have me as her nurse "for real next time." Hearing this little girl have the upmost faith in me as a professional before I could even see it was an astounding moment of my life.

Haley Anders. BSN, RN

He Was My Very First Patient

It was in my first semester clinical, Strategies for Professional Nursing. It was my first clinical day; first day as a nurse. I was excited. I was assigned a nearby hospital with our professor. I had heard great things about her and was about to find out first hand why she was such a spectacular nurse. I was assigned by her to a patient at the very end of the long hallway. He was my first patient and that day was special. I entered the room to see what I could do for him. He was on bed rest. He was a large man. In his room were pictures hanging of his son. I began to speak with him. He had dementia, but spoke to me without any indications of it. He had been flown in from another area due to Hurricane Katrina. It was Monday and he seemed upset. He wasn't feeling well and was in pain. I felt bad for him. His sheets at the end of the bed were a little bloody. His feet had been elevated but were now resting on the bed. His concern became my concern. My professor entered the room and she brought sunshine. Right away, the patient began to sob like a little boy as he told her about his feet and pain. Obtaining booties for his feet seemed like an ongoing battle he was facing. It seemed as though it would take an act from Congress to get new booties for his feet. She comforted him, held his hand, and sincerely listened to him. I really appreciated her compassion. That is why I want to be a nurse. Being a nurse is about showing compassion to people. When people are enduring their hardest times in life, I want to be there to help lift them up. I want to bring them hope. My professor assured the patient she would get new booties for his feet today. She came through with her promise. Often times, when I would see that hospital as I walked to or from my car to school or the hospital, I would think of that man at the end of the hallway, alone, on bed rest in his hospital room. As a nurse, I will serve tirelessly, love unconditionally, and hope endlessly.

Andrea (Johnson) Auman, BSN, RN

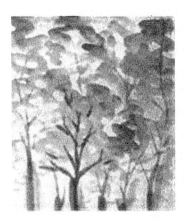

My True Calling in Nursing

I realized that a career in nursing was my true calling while caring for an ailing elderly woman stricken with the late stages of lymphoma. With all the strength and vitality she could possibly muster, she somehow managed to greet me with a robust and soulful "Hi, Meja!" As I entered her room to administer her medications and perform my assessments, her tired eyes would light up and her face seemed to glow. "How are you doing today?" I asked my fragile patient. "Ay, Meja," she answered. "I'm so weak and so tired. Even after sleeping all night long I am still so very tired." I conversed earnestly with my patient while diligently performing my assessment, then sat quietly at her bedside while she enjoyed breakfast.

Gazing empathetically at my patient, I couldn't help but reflect on my own familial experiences with cancer, most recently a family member, who was afflicted with renal cell carcinoma. .I remembered that some of the most critical aspects of that person's road to recovery included simple things, such as a helping hand, a listening ear, a sincere and caring heart and lots of love. We incorporated other integrative modalities of healing such as music therapy and walking outdoors in the sunshine.

Recalling these moments encouraged me to slow down and take time to genuinely listen to my patient. She was lonely, afraid and desperate for somebody—anybody—to keep her company. I joyfully obliged, and remembered that I chose nursing so that I could lovingly serve others, believing that when we serve others, we are also serving God. As nurses, we will never look back fondly at memories of hurried care that was delivered hastily and half-heartedly. However, as healers and stewards of the human spirit, nurses will never regret the great moments in which we offered a shoulder to cry on, and a quiet moment of simply "being with" our patients. The spirit of nursing calls us to the service of humanity through our unique gifts of love, compassion and presence.

Theresa M. Ballard, BSN, RN

A Patient's Poem

A patient that made me realize that I had chosen the right profession was a man in his nineties who was a WWII veteran. What makes this patient so special to me is because he started telling me what he believed makes a good nurse from his many years of dealing with them. He was open about his past experiences with nurses. He mentioned that one of the most important things that I had to do as a new nurse was to check on my patients as soon as my shift started. He told me that during one of his previous hospital stays, he experienced a 3-hour lapse between the time that the night shift nurse said goodbye and the morning nurse introduced himself/herself to the patient. Another memory of this patient was when he needed to get a cardiac ultrasound done. The patient requested for me to stay in the room because he was scared of the procedure

I was able to establish a good rapport with him. Within the two days that I took care of him, he told me many stories about his life. I shared some of my feelings with him as well. I felt we connected not only by the stories we told, but with our military service too. During the last day, I mentioned to him that we had a big test coming up the same week. He told me that my classmates and I had nothing to worry about and that we were going to do well. He then gave me a poem to remember.

> Now that I lay me down to study,
> I pray the Lord I won't go nutty.
> If I should fail to learn this junk
> I pray the Lord I will not flunk.
>
> But if I do, don't pity me at all;
> Just lay my bones down in the study hall.
> Tell my teachers I did my best,
> Then pile the books upon my chest

Now I lay me down to rest,
And pray I'll pass tomorrow's test.
If I should die before I wake
That's one less test I'll have to take.

    Anonymous (given to the student by his patient)

Leonardo X. Bermudez, BSN, RN

A Wonderful Experience

I had a wonderful experience on my first Leadership and Management clinical day. A particular patient truly touched my heart and made me realize that the hospital is my "home." I have always been drawn to nursing and enjoy caring for others. I find satisfaction in knowing that I provided the best possible care to my patient (through physical tasks and emotional support). Communication is an easy endeavor, when approached in a sincere manner. My patients appreciate the time given (if only a few minutes), to sit down and discuss their concerns or needs. This patient, which I would like to focus my discussion, had many cultural desires. He had moved here from another country and although his English was impressive, he still needed help expressing his needs. Communication is an essential element of medical care. I wonder how many patients are able to seek care in the United States, without the aid of an advocate or translator. We had wonderful conversations, about his life in the US. We discussed his job, family, illness, and even sports! He has a passion for baseball. I was able to relate because I played softball as a child. A true connection was made when I held his hand during a procedure. This simple act made him feel comfortable and safe. He couldn't stand the sight of blood and we talked through the procedure. He didn't even notice the pain! I felt we "bonded" and was honestly sad to leave for the day. He had a big grin on his face and told my nurse. "She's gonna be a great nurse." This impression has merely amplified my desire to understand other languages. I continue to try to become fluent in Spanish with an added appreciation of its worth. Regardless of nationality, disability, or age, it is imperative to treat every individual with the proper respect and dignity.

Kristen Cannon, BSN, RN

A Great Patient

As I introduce myself to a patient, I always smile and try to get a feel for the situation. I try to determine the patient's' outlook on their condition. I had been assigned to a unit in which, as a student, I was unfamiliar and uncomfortable. I gowned up and entered the patient's room. I smiled and said "Hello" to Roger, the patient. He was a very small gentleman diagnosed with throat cancer. Roger had been through many procedures to get rid of the cancer, which seemed to be never ending. He had a tracheostomy and no voice box. His throat has an incision bilaterally, and he had many complications in between. In my opinion, Roger was in bad shape, but he always smiled and nodded. Although he could not talk to me, he found ways to get the point across. He wrote or used hand gestures. He was a very pleasant man to be around, especially considering his situation, and he never complained. After watching Roger and his situation over the next three weeks, I was able to learn so much. Not only did Roger have a positive attitude about life and his condition, he had the drive to get better. He wanted to go home. I enjoyed the emotional aspect of nursing as well as the scientific or pathologic side too. Roger had some very rare complications that left me asking questions every day. As I followed Roger's case, I found that learning is never fully accomplished. I was not the only one scratching my head. The other nurses, along with doctors and surgeons, were also quite perplexed with some of the conditions that arose in Roger's case. I do not know whatever happened to Roger, but he was a great patient. He united a team of medical professionals and showed me that sometimes even the best of the best are not going to know the answers, but we keep trying.

As a nursing student, I was inspired by Roger to ask questions, learn more, and fully engage as part of the healthcare team.

Laura L.Carey, BSN, RN

*This patient's name was changed for patient confidentially.

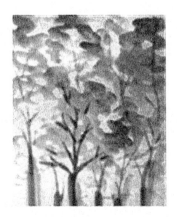

A Patient I Won't Forget

There have been many different patients that I have taken care of that have had an impact on the way I view myself in my nursing career but none more than the patient that I had in my Chronic Clinical class third semester. It was a Spanish speaking patient who just wanted a blanket, and she was so thankful it made me feel good. As my nurse and I worked on taking care of her, she saw our teamwork and what we were doing for her. She gave both my nurse and me a "WOW" card. This is a card that patients can fill out when they feel they have received excellent care. I was so excited. I was just doing my job but yet to her it was a whole lot more. I never felt more appreciated, and it was very rewarding to help someone and have them appreciate it. I think at that point I believed that I chose the right career path. I may have bad days, but I can always think about that patient and the situation that she was in and optimism she had. I will never forget, and it will always cheer me up. I think that nursing is a great field to go into and as we practice nursing there is going to be many different situations that can get us flustered, irritated, or even made, but when we help make lives better and see the smile on the patients face by helping them, all the negative emotions will go away.

Charles Chaiya, BSN, RN

Patient Impact in Nursing

It was another day filled with nerves and excitement as I arrived on the unit. Once meeting up with the nurse I was assigned to follow, we went to received report. As the departing nurse gave us report, she mentioned that one of the patients' spoke only Spanish. The nurse I was following gave me an apprehensive look. I told her not to worry because I spoke Spanish. After hearing the report given by the departing nurse, I was interested in learning more about the patient's case. As I walked into the patient's room, I braced myself with confidence and a smiling face. I introduced the nurse and myself to the patient and continued with the assessment. My patient suffered from a terrible infection on her breast. The orange peel appeared as they described in nursing school, but it did not prepare me for what I was about to witness. As I removed the top layer of the dressing, I witnessed a very large incision. The patient was in a somber mood. Not only was she in tremendous physical pain, she was also experiencing separation anxiety from her baby. Her baby was a 3-week old little girl that was being watched by a family member. As I was in the patient's room, she informed me that she had been breastfeeding, but shortly after started feeling ill and experiencing fever. The reason she postponed seeking care was because she did not have insurance. Delay of care is an enormous issue for patients that do not have insurance. It was difficult for me not to feel sympathetic towards the patient's situation. The nurse informed me that we were going to have to change the patient's wound dressing. She also expressed the excessive amount of pain the patient would undergo due to the process. The nurse wanted me to translate the step-by-step process to the patient's husband because he was going to be changing the dressing at home. Prior to the dressing change, the nurse gave the patient pain medication to help with pain during the process of the change. The nurse and I gathered all the materials needed to complete the dressing change. As the nurse began to strip away the top layer of the dressing the patient was tense and terrified. Once the nurse started gently pulling the gauze out of the incision, the patient's face turned pale. The patient reached her hand to me. I held the patient's hand and coached her during the procedure as tears ran down her face. The thought of having the patient's husband accomplishing the dressing change at home seemed unrealistic.

At this time, the reality of care the hospital provides for an uninsured patient played out. It seemed outrageous that a patient with a huge open incision would be going home. Upon discharging the patient, I explained the importance of taking her medication and changing her dressing. That's when the patient told me that she did not have the money or the resource to buy the medication and gauze. I told the nurse and we were able to gather some materials she can take home. As for the medications, the nurse and I involved the charge nurse. The charge nurse was able to go to the pharmacist and filled the antibiotic prescription. If we were not able to get the materials for the dressing change or the antibiotics, the patient would just return to the hospital in a worse condition. The gratitude that the patient expressed was extremely fulfilling. I might have not cured her or taken away the pain, but I was there to hold her hand and help get her the necessary materials she needed. After that experience, I knew that nursing was the right profession for me. I was able to impact a patient's life for the better and for that I am grateful.

Charisa Chavez, BSN, RN

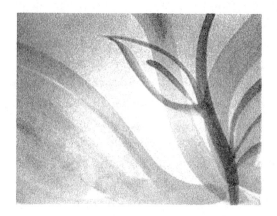

A Patient To Remember

There have been many patients I have had the pleasure of caring for that reassured me that I had to be a nurse. One man in particular I will always remember. Even as I sit here writing, I get choked up and teary eyed remembering him. He is the reason why I know I'm a nurse and not just a person who is trying to do their job. During my first clinical, a night shift as a matter of fact, in my first semester of nursing school, I had Mr. X as a patient. Mr. X was a new lower extremity amputee, who had diabetes, and on contact precaution for MRSA. He was experiencing phantom limb syndrome, very scared, confused, and worried. I was able to complete patient care with him, but the most I knew I could do for him was give him my company. For my first day our instructor just wanted us to have one patient, so I took advantage of the moments. I had nothing to do and just sat with this man.

Upon talking to Mr. X, I discovered that he loved to paint and draw. It was something we held in common. We exchanged techniques, ideas, and spoke as through we were old pals. At one point I realized Mr. X was no longer complaining of pain. I knew he didn't have pain because we were speaking of something he obviously had passion for and was distracted. I noticed he had a pencil, which he was using for a cross word puzzle book. I asked him if he ever drew when he was upset or sad, because I knew that I used times when I was filled with emotion to create my art. I explained that times of emotion bring out my best work and it also helps to calm me down and come to more tranquil state of mind. It distracts me, and I explained that it could probably help him with his pain and also bring out some very expressive creativity. He told me, "You know what, I never thought of it way. Now that I think about it I do draw to distract myself. Someone will get me mad and I draw. I think my mom, who passed away, and I drew. Wow, I do use that. Plus I'll have something to do." So I went and asked the nurse if I could have some computer paper for my patient. Mr. X began drawing right away. He first started off sketching a caricature of me. He then drew a picture that was in a magazine. In the middle of drawing, Mr. X started crying. I immediately asked him he was having pain. He said, "No, meja. I'm not in pain." He paused for a bit and continued. "Just real happy. You know since I've been here with the MRSA I feel like I haven't been treated like a human being, but instead like some infected animal that had to be put away and separated from the rest of the world. And you're here keeping me company and helping me. While it seems like everyone else is in such a rush to get out of the room and you're just here with me. Thank you. You're not a student anymore. Meja you're a nurse and a real good person." A couple of tears ran down my face and even though this man was on contact precautions I still continued to treat him as a human being as he said. He reached out to hug me and I hugged him back in my gown, gloves, and all.

Later on in the day his wife came to visit. Shortly after entering his room she can out asking for me. I thought Mr. X needed something. The nurse showed her who I was. She came to me and said. "You know this is the first time in days that I have finally been able to see my real husband again. He told me what you did. You brought some life back to him. Thank you Meja" and she gave me a big hug. They didn't know it was my first day. A week later in lecture we learned about alternative medicine and treatments. Drawing was mentioned; I smiled and remembered Mr. X. Until this day I still remember Mr. X, and I am proud of being a nurse.

April Cortinas, BSN, RN

An Apology

I knew I was meant to be a nurse when I was caring for a patient in the intensive care unit. His diagnosis was "chest pain." Upon assessment, it was discovered this individual was in kidney failure and was suffering from an exacerbation of Hepatitis. This patient had been using the Emergency Department as his primary care as he was uninsured and was homeless. He had frequented many of the hospitals and was known for his extended stays.

As I began to do an assessment on him while giving him a bed bath, he became belligerent with me, raising his voice and cursing at me. It was then I leaned in and looked him in the eyes and told him that I was there to help him get better. I told him that I would treat him the way I would want to be treated, that I was there for him. Within minutes he began to cry. He then told me, "You don't understand, I haven't had anyone look at me as though I am person in a long time. Everyone looks at me as though I am trash. My own mother won't even speak to me. I have nobody. You are the first person that has been nice to me, and I know you are trying to help me. I'm sorry for what I said earlier."

I spent the remainder of my shift with this individual. Knowing that I not only was there that day to assist in the healing of his body, but hopefully also his heart confirmed I was in the right profession. To make a difference in someone's life, no matter how big or small, this is success

Christina Cunningham, BSN, RN

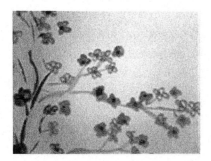

Comeback Kid

My First day in the ICU was an exciting one, and I was ready for anything except for the patient that I was assigned. I got report that morning along with my nurse. It was a teenage boy who had been in a motor vehicle collision (MVC) with an open abdominal wound, a splenectomy and partial liver removal. The patient had coded 5 times in the ER and 3 times in the ICU, and had received multiple units of blood. In my mind all I could think was *alright let's see how today goes.*

Then I walked into the room. Seeing him was completely different from what I had heard. Before that day I had never been in an ICU, let alone been with such a critical patient. The room was quiet and still with just the background noises of beeping and the swishing of his ventilator which seemed to fade away as I walked in the room. Who was he? What had happened to him? It was early in the morning so no one was visiting yet. The nurse came in with a handful of tasks we needed to complete before the family came in so I focused on that at the time. I was completely overwhelmed with every line, the ventilator, and the amount of medicine hanging in the bags over him. He was in an induced coma and was jaundice with a distended belly covered with a wound vac the size of open magazine. His body was still swollen and bruised from the trauma he suffered. He wasn't expected to make it, but he did. Eventually his mother arrived. I could tell she was nervous because the nurse caring for her son in his fragile condition was not one he had before. There was definitely a tension in the room the entire day. Every task I performed was like I was being watched by a mama bear looking over her defenseless cub, and I could feel her eyes on me the entire time. I understood completely where she was coming from and didn't have a problem with it. I had the same patient the following day but with a nurse that mom loved and trusted. Everything was different that day and the entire feeling was better. I got to talk to mom and shared some stories with her and vice-versa. My nurse also had confidence in me, and I learned a lot from him. I can't really explain how great that feels.

I had the same patient the following week for two more days with the same nurse. I learned more, and my patient began to progress little by little. The rest of that semester I felt inclined to see how he was doing and made time to go see him and his mother. One week he was off the paralytic. The next he was awake and aware enough he could trace people with his eyes. I went the following couple weeks to see him watching TV and acknowledging commands. It was like a miracle before my eyes. He was never out of the woods. But he kept getting better, and I always seemed to be there for another miraculous event. Once he was able to communicate with everyone, I went and visited. He didn't like my jokes very much and probably thought, "Who is this lady?" because most of the time I cared for him he was asleep. Eventually he began to know me, and he, his mom and family appreciated the fact that I did care. I really don't know why this patient and his family touched me so, but they did. Maybe it was the fact that I witnessed a miracle before my own eyes or how incredible his mother was and how she kept it together for him and the rest of her family. I hope that I have more experiences like this as begin to practice as an RN. I'm happy to report that he's doing well and on a very long road to recovery, nicknamed the Comeback Kid.

Carla Dearinger, BSN, RN

Miracle of Birth

I don't have kids, so the "miracle of birth" feeling isn't something I can directly relate to. Don't get me wrong I love babies and want to have one someday, but to me the actual labor and delivery process seemed sort of frightening and dare I say, gross. Before entering nursing school, I had heard stories of stitches, stretching, and tearing in places I didn't know possible. Once I got into nursing school, the process was explained and it all almost became normal to me, until the day I actually had to watch it. I walked into my clinical and immediately found out I was going to see a natural birth. I was excited and nervous at the same time. Through our classes, I knew what to expect but this was a stranger. After meeting my patient, I felt reassured that this would be a good experience as this was her third child and she felt very confident and ready to have the baby. Only five minutes had gone by when the baby decided to make its entrance, and watching it was the complete opposite of what I expected. It was so beautiful. I couldn't believe how much I was wrong about birth. In that moment I realized how much I wanted to be a nurse and help bring babies into the world. I loved how my patient handled her birth, no screaming or crying, just doing what came natural to her to deliver her baby into the world. It was a great experience.

Gillian DeMase, BSN, RN

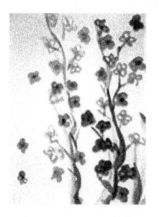

A Most Inspiring Patient

The most inspiring patient I remember was a man who I only got to take care of for a brief eight hours. He was recently downgraded from the Cardiac Intensive Care Unit (ICU) onto the telemetry flour, where I was taking care of him after his second heart attack and first code. He was a 58 year old male with a wife of 25 years and 2 daughters around my age, overall a family much like my own. After doing my health assessment on him, I asked him about his recent hospital stay, and he was more than willing to tell me whatever I wanted to hear. He told me about how he had grown up in San Antonio, and being Hispanic never had a very good diet. He exercised some, but just enough to keep his weight in check. After learning about his family and his life's work he started to focus on his health.

He had his first heart attack five years ago. It was a very mild one and he counted himself lucky but didn't really change much about his lifestyle. This time around, he told me, *"was a completely different story."* The way he described it was: sometimes it takes almost dying to make you realize something needs to change. He then told me about all the different things he had been learning about that he can change to prevent this from happening again. He said that before these past couple of days, he didn't really have much faith in doctors or healthcare, but "something about them bringing you back from death, gives you as different perspective."

Knowing that my profession was able to give this man even one more day with this wife and daughters helps reassure me that nursing is the way to go. Being able to provide this patient with the information he needed to start bettering his life makes it all worth it.

Natalie Deuel, BSN, RN

School Experience

One of my most memorable experiences during nursing school that made me happy that I was entering the profession of nursing, happened during my first semester as a student. The patient that I was helping was a male admitted to the hospital for a cardio vascular accident. While providing his care throughout the day he was very determined to do his activities of daily living (ADL's) without assistance but because he was weak on his left side, he needed assistance with 90 percent of his tasks. He was a memorable patient because he showed an appreciation for my help by verbally thanking me for helping him while allowing him to maintain his dignity. This made me smile inside because, even though I was selflessly helping someone else, he appreciated my efforts even though I was only a first semester student who had very limited nursing skills.

Yashika Denise Edwards, BSN, RN

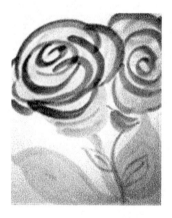

A Patient's Fears

During the fall semester, I had a patient on the telemetry unit. She was my patient for four clinical days. I had established a relationship with her over these four days. She was very polite and always pleasant to be around. My last day with her was the Monday before Thanksgiving. She was upset because her family had not come to visit her in the hospital. They called to ask her if she could still cook all the food for Thanksgiving dinner. She was very frustrated that their only concern was Thanksgiving dinner.

Later that day I was in the nurse's station and the secretary told me that one of my patients was asking for me. As I entered the room, I found my patient crying in her bed. I asked her to tell me what she was crying about. She said the doctor's had just come in and told her she was going down for some operation. She was very scared and did not understand what the doctors were going to do to her. I brought her some tissues and sat and spoke with her about her procedure. We discussed her fears about the procedure, and I asked if she wanted to speak with the doctors again before her procedure. She said yes so I had them paged. Before I left that day she gave me a big hug and thanked me for being so understanding. She said that she was so thankful to have me as her nurse. I will never forget her because that was the day I truly felt like I had made a difference in a patient's life.

Julie Engle, BSN, RN

Confirmation

I realized the moment I met Samantha* that I was in the right place for the right reasons. Samantha had just had her first baby and was a little nervous about being a new mom. She had planned her pregnancy out and taken classes to prepare herself and husband for what was to come. All the planning and preparation had paid off throughout her pregnancy and delivery; however, now that she had her baby, she didn't plan that breastfeeding would be so difficult.

I was assigned Samantha as my postpartum patient and was a bit bummed about not being in Labor and Delivery (L&D), which I just loved. I had to now handle the "not-so glamorous" part of Obstetrics (OB) and was dreading it. I walked in to assess her and get started with my nursing care when I noticed Samantha struggling with getting baby to latch-on. I asked if I could help her and she was immediately relieved that I was there. I was able to reposition her and baby and instruct Samantha on proper latching and positioning techniques that would facilitate breastfeeding. I ended up sitting with her and teaching her for about an hour and walked out feeling more fulfilled and rewarded than at any other time in nursing school.

I went and checked on Samantha and her baby about an hour later. She had just put the baby back down so she and baby could rest. Samantha told me that she had not slept since she gave birth due to her worrying about not being able to feed her baby. She thanked me and told me that she was glad that she could now rest knowing that she will be able to continue using the techniques we worked on to breastfeed. She also mentioned that breastfeeding was extremely important to her and that other nurses were merely suggesting that she just give formula to her baby without putting some time in to help her breastfeed.

My experiences with Samantha, other postpartum patients, as well as with my overall love of L&D, solidified my passion to be an OB nurse. There is no question in my mind where I belong. I believe the feeling of peace and fulfillment in this area will help me be an even better nurse that I could possibly be anywhere else. I definitely made the right choice in wanting to be a nurse, and more specifically an OB nurse

Tammy Evans, BSN, RN

The patient's name was changed to protect patient confidentially.

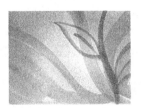

Confirmation Of My Chosen Path As An RN

Over the course of my nurses training I have encountered many patients. As I sit and reflect over the past four semesters, I find it difficult to find just one patient who confirmed my reason for being a registered nurse, I have taken a little something from each patient that said I'm exactly where I want to be. This last semester has truly confirmed that I chose the right profession.

One patient comes to mind to confirm that decision. He was a patient who was pretty much written off as "going to die by the end of my shift", as the RN assigned to him commented. He had a cerebral hemorrhage. He wasn't my patient the first week, but I still talked to him and looked after him. I just couldn't understand how the RN could "write him off". She paid very little attention to him. I just wouldn't give up on him that easily. He was non-verbal and just laid there with vacant eyes. He had bilateral paresis of the upper and lower extremities. No one visited him at first, so the tech and I were the only ones interacting with him, except for the doctors on rounds. I greeted him by name when I came into the room. I assisted the tech in giving him a bath. She interacted with him and talked to him like any other patient. I left after day two not knowing whether I would come back and find him.

The following Monday I walked into the room and there he was. His once vacant eyes literally lit up. There was no mistaking it. For me that little bit of recognition told me he was truly "still in there." I can't describe how that made me feel. I greeted him with a smile and performed my assessment. He reacted to pain when his extremities were barely moved. I talked to him, and apologized when I caused him discomfort. At this stage it was just basic skills. Giving meds, flushing his IV, checking his fluids and TPN as he was NPO, turning every two hours, neuro checks every four hours, etc.

The next day his eyes signaled recognition again. He was no longer NPO. He whispered his name when I asked him to tell me. The physical therapist and I talked to him while performing passive range of motion exercises. I fed him thickened liquids for breakfast, which he drank as though he just walked through the desert. His nephew came to visit and then his niece. They expressed concern. I engaged them in conversation about how well he was doing, while talking "with him" instead of "about him". Later when he shivered, I asked if he was cold and he whispered, "Yes". Lunchtime was great. When asked, he indicated his preference for sweet potatoes over mashed potatoes with a mod. He had Ensure and I assisted in giving him small sips with a straw. He weekly took his left hand and grabbed the can and gently brought it and the straw to his lips and drank. I was so happy and praised him so much. It was unbelievable! I made it a point to tell his docs.

That is why I do what I do. It is because against all odds, the human spirit and the will to live is evident everyday on the floor. The fact that I may have made a little bit of difference; I don't even want to take credit for because it took teamwork with others who saw the person not the patient. But it sure makes me feel good to have been a part of it! I know not all my patients will recover fully. I was able to be a part of one who passed from this life to another. But even there I found satisfaction in the privilege of caring for another who needed it. I have truly found my calling.

Karen B. Fulton, BSN, RN

Personal Narrative

During my time in nursing school, I have had many opportunities to work with patients in the hospital through my clinicals. I will never forget the first patient I ever had my first semester in nursing school. I feel like working with the first patient really helped me as a student to see that I was in the right profession.

Even though our clinical group did not get the same experiences initially with working in a hospital setting, we still were able to practice the basics of nursing and get comfortable talking with our patients. My first patient was an elderly female who had lived in the assisted living area for a while, but came to our floor because of a hip fracture from a fall. When I met this patient, she was in the process of healing and had a positive outlook with getting back to adequate health. As I began to just talk with her, she told me about all her stories in life and how she was a famous dancer on a popular television show. Her life was so interesting and I enjoyed the moments I had just listening to her. Although this event was not something exciting like saving a life, it was influential in my career because it helped me to see that being a nurse was not just helping people to get better. It was being there for a person when they possibly need it the most. From then on I realized that I knew I had chosen the right profession

Jacob Garcia, BSN, RN

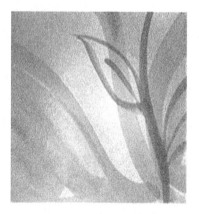

That One Patient

I was in my second semester of nursing school doing my chronic rotation on a medical-surgical unit. I had a Spanish speaking female patient who recently had a colostomy placed. I remember her being very embarrassed and crying when we had to change out the bag or when gas was released from the colostomy. I knew that she couldn't understand me, so I tried showing as much empathy as I could with my actions. I gave her a very thorough bed bath, rubbed her feet with lotion, and brushed her hair (the simple things that we are taught to do that I didn't think much about at the time.) Her husband came in a little after lunch time, so I gave them their privacy for a while. After speaking to his wife, he came up to me in the hallway and asked me to come in to see his wife. I didn't know that her husband spoke very good English. I thought she needed something, so I followed him into the room. She started talking to him in Spanish, and he began to translate for her. She told me that the care I provided her and how I approached her made her feel special and that I was a gift from God. She said many other things that made me feel like I had done more than my job, and I truly felt blessed to be a nurse. I left the hospital that day thinking I had really done something to help a patient and to better her outcome. That was a day that I really knew that I had picked the right profession.

Jessica Garrison, BSN, RN

Voices of the Voiceless

Ventilators: Machines designed to keep a client ventilated. This was a mysterious piece of equipment added to the endless list of "need to know" items as I prepared for my rotation in ICU. The settings, the abbreviated names for functions of the machine and the measurements of client response were whirling in my mind as I walked into the Pediatric Intensive Care Unit (PICU) for the first time.

No previous experience of my baby boomer life prepared me for the sight of the five year old girl being treated for injuries sustained in a senseless motor vehicle accident. Her face and hands were puffy from retained fluids. Her hair was still matted with blood which an attentive PICU nurse had attempted to clean during the night. The metal clips kept her hair parted in a horseshoe shape across her skull. Her right arm was in a cast up to the elbow with puffy little fingers protruding from the edge. Chest tubes were making their entrance into her smooth, brown chest wall in four places. Of course, a "Foley" catheter continuously drained her bladder. Her right femoral artery was the site of the arterial line which gave the staff access to her blood and it's gases. IV fluids pumped into her fevered body through the catheter in her left wrist. The ventilator, the machine that I had been studying the previous day, was in place behind the head of the bed. Set to deliver 50 percent oxygen, it was keeping those child lungs inflated and maintaining a blood oxygen level adequate for sustaining life and promote healing. The machine continuously pumped, down the flexible tubing and down into the endotracheal tube fixated in her throat. She was unable to independently push air into or out of her lungs. She was voiceless.

I felt I was invading this child's privacy as I made my way to the bedside to assess her physical status. She was unresponsive to voice command although I noticed an upper body response to touch. Her native language was not my native language, but I felt compelled to speak to her in soft tones and call her name often as I completed the assessment. Eye contact was not possible as hers remained swollen closed. Morphine keep her calm.

This picture is all wrong! My heart wrenched as I looked at her still body. Children should be playing in the park, laughing and shouting with life and energy. I cried inside knowing this was the result of a senseless choice of an irresponsible parent. My hope returns as I realize I can be an instrument of her healing. As I speak and assess and check fluid levels and pray, I choose to believe she will have an opportunity to recover fully and regain her childhood. Nursing is part of the restorative process given to us by our Creator. How blessed I am to be able to participate in this work.

Mary Jane Gillespie, BSN, RN

Giving Comfort

I wanted a vocation in nursing to help people; to help fix people. On my first clinical day during my first semester, my first patient wasn't able to be fixed. He was on hospice and actively dying. The day prior had been his last to eat or drink so the nurses told me he would be gone soon. This went against everything that I had in mind. Starry-eyed, I believed that with cups of pills and an expertly filled cup of ice water, I could help heal the sick. From my first patient, I realized it wasn't always about healing but about comforting. There was no health history taken or questions asked, it was hand holding and oral swabs to help moisten his cracked lips. There were no "thank you's" but rather looking into thankful eyes that knew more than my own. At the end of the day, I looked at my cohorts who had gotten to practice skills. They passed meds and helped with patients' activities of daily living and had things to brag about. I, on the other hand, had only the memory of my first patient, who taught me it isn't all about fixing people, but about giving comfort during the worst days.

Elizabeth Gorychka, BSN, RN

A Patient Remembered

I remember all of the patients I have taken care of in nursing school, and I really don't think one has stood out to me for a particular reason. I do know that with several of these patients there has been one thing in common that makes me realize nursing is the right profession for me. It is those patients, and I would say about 75 percent of those I have taken care of, with whom I have had meaningful conversations and connections. Even those patients that can't communicate at all or very well, such as those with dementia, patients in the psychiatric ward, babies in the nursery, patients that only speak Spanish, and even patients in comas, I feel I have made connections with them or helped them in a way that made me feel good at the end of the day. The emotional, personal, and teaching side of nursing is what I love.

During my nursing school experience, I have seen life brought into this world, held and rocked babies that are hungry and sleepy, given them their first bath, comforted babies born with addictions, and helped a mother to breastfeed for the first time. I have talked to teens about sex, birth control, self-esteem, depression, suicide, and making less risky choices. I've talked to adults about living a healthier lifestyle as far as nutrition and exercise, what to do about their alcohol addition, living with your partner and AIDS, how to keep track of medications, and the list goes on and on. I have talked with patients about their fear of dying. I have seen my patient die, and I have talked to families after death of a loved one. I have talked with and listened to patients that are speaking nonsense as with dementia, patients with psychiatric issues, and ICU syndrome.

Regardless of the things I have seen or the skills I have done, what makes me know nursing is the right profession for me is the satisfaction I get from helping someone who is completely dependent on me, listening to someone who just needs someone to talk to, or just getting a patient to smile. I have had a few patients tell me, "Thank you for caring about me, no one else here acts like they do. You will be a great nurse." And then they hold my hand of hug me. I love knowing that I have made someone's day a little nicer when they need it most, or knowing that something we talked about may impact them today or the rest of their lives. I'm thankful for the experiences with these patients, and I hope I have touched them as much as they have touched me.

Andrea Greer, BSN, RN

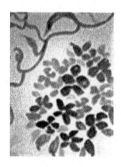

A Man Who Made a Lasting Impression

During my clinical experience, I met a man who was admitted with abdominal pain and distention. He was very uncomfortable, and in the early stages of his treatment I was at a loss as to how I could help. Throughout my clinical rotation, this man was in the hospital. I saw him get better, and then have setbacks. But then he kept getting better and better. He was in the hospital for a while, and I got to know him fairly well. He talked a lot about his culture, where he was from, and his family. I loved learning from him. He and his family were always so appreciative of the care that he received.

As the patient continued to improve, his discharge was imminent and his time in the hospital was coming to an end. It was amazing to see his transformation – a real metamorphosis – from the man with extreme abdominal pain and distention to the pleasant man that just wanted me to stay in his room and care for him. Isn't that what this job is about? I think people forget that we all went into this profession because we care. This man and his gentle, kind spirit made a lasting impression on me in my journey through nursing school because he showed me how we really can impact people through simple acts of genuine kindness. And for that, I will always be grateful.

Sara Hajda, BSN, RN

A Simple Conversation

Today I realized I made the right chose to enter in the nursing profession. I really enjoy talking with people and getting to know them. Before starting nursing school, I really wanted to become a nurse and work with pregnant women, whether that be well-clinic, antepartum, intrapartum, or postpartum. Since going through that rotation, I know that is the avenue I still want to pursue. But today I made a connection with a patient who was not assigned to me. He was walking the halls and out of politeness I asked how he was doing. He replied find and asked how I was doing. Our conversation took a life of its own as we walked down the hall together. In that short period of time, I learned so much about this man: where he was born, what he did for a living, what he dreamed of doing, his children and grandchildren. We made our way back to his room and parted ways. He genuinely thanked me for taking the time to walk with him; and that's when it hit me. I am in the right profession. I am here to do the little things that others may neglect or not have time to do. I am here to gain insight about the people in our society, to form a connection and learn from them.

Krystal (Wohlfahrt) Henk. BSN, RN

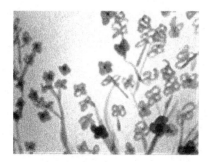

My Most Memorable Patient

As I was thinking about which patient I wanted to write about for this assignment I always kept coming back to the same one. This patient always stands out to me as someone who reminded me that nursing is about caring for the patient. The simple things we do for our patients are the things that can make the biggest difference for them.

This patient had been in the hospital for a number of weeks and was going to be there for at least another month. She was in a private room and her family only visited every other weekend because she was from a town that was at least a two hour drive away. From a medical perspective this patient did not need a lot. She was there more for observation and monitoring of her condition. Throughout my day on this unit I had mostly spent time helping with things like vital signs and assisting patients with activities. When the nurse I was with asked me if I wanted to help this patient go outside for a little while, I thought, "Sure, no big deal." So I got a wheelchair and helped her into it. Before going outside she asked if she could go see another unit in the hospital that she would be moving to in a few weeks. So I took her up there, and since I was familiar with the unit, I showed her around and let her see where everything was located. Then we went outside and set in a breezeway for about 30 minutes and talked. We didn't really talk about anything important. It was just an opportunity to sit outside for a few minutes. After about 30 minutes we went back inside and I helped the patient back into bed and went on with my day.

I left that unit that day thinking I had not really done much for my patients from a nursing perspective, but my instructor later told me that the nurse commented how much I had done to help this one patient. It didn't occur to me at first but then I realized that by taking the time to help her I made an impact in her day. She might not have gotten to go outside or go see the other unit and certainly would not have gotten 30 minutes to just sit and talk with someone.

This patient reminded me that nursing is not just about the skills. I wanted to become a nurse to help care for people and my experience with this patient reminded me of that. We have the opportunity to do so much more for our patients than just perform skills and administer medications; we can truly make a difference even if it is just by assisting them outside for a few minutes.

Kelly Hines, BSN, RN

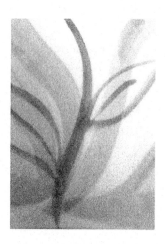

Paralyzed

It was a day like any other day. The sun was rising, wind was gently blowing through the trees, and leaves were dancing along the sidewalk. Not expecting to see much today, I grudgingly walked toward the hospital. Little did I know today would be a day that changed my life.

My clinical group met in the lobby and my instructor handed us all our assignments. I went straight to my unit. The day was slow. But I followed my nurse and took advantage of any opportunity I could, like a respectable nursing student should. Then it happened - "code blue on the floor!" I was shocked. I had never witnessed a code before. Paralyzed with fear, I looked up to see flashes of dark blue and green rushing past me and into the room right beside me. My patient was coding, and here I stood, not knowing what I, as a first-semester nursing student, could do.

I turned to the room and witnessed a chaotic scene. A giant crowd of people was stuffed into one tiny room. My nurse was over the bed bagging the patient, while another nurse was well in the middle of compressions, and another nurse was carefully taking notes on the side. I tried to sneak in for a better look, but the crash cart nearly blocked the entire door. Before I knew it, everything was over and the patient was revived. My nurse and I took my patient and moved her to another room to stabilize her. That ended my clinical day.

On the drive back to my house, I looked back on the events of the day and realized something. I want to do that. I want to save lives. I want to be confident enough to know what to do in these situations. I don't want to run away; I want to run towards. I don't want fear to paralyze me; I want faith to push me forward. I want to do something for this world. That day, I realized I *truly* want to be a nurse.

Jenny Idicula, BSN, RN

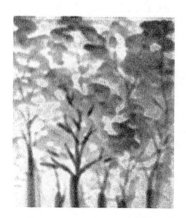

Brief Paragraph

Throughout my clinical experience in nursing school there have been multiple patients that have made me realize that I am in the right profession. However, there is one patient in particular that showed me that my hard work and helpfulness was greatly appreciated. I took care of this patient my first week in Leadership and Management Clinical. She was the sweetest lady that I have ever met. She had been in the hospital through Christmas Day, New Year's, and her birthday. Her son visited her often but was not there when I provided care, so I went into the patient's room from time to time just to talk with her and keep her company.

During the day, the patient had expressed to me the care that she had been receiving throughout her hospital stay, and it was very upsetting to hear. She was telling me that the night nurse did not treat her well. I was listening while she expressed her feelings to let her know that I was there for her. Unlike her impression of the night nurse, I provided professional nursing care and showed respect for the patient. I went in the room almost every hour to talk with her.

After my shift was over I went into the patient's room to let her know that I was leaving, and she made a very nice comment as I was walking out of the room. The patient turned to the respiratory therapist who was in her room and told her that I was the sweetest girl. Her comment made me realize that I have the qualities of a nurse and knowing that I could be there for the patient during this vulnerable time makes me want to be the best nurse I can be. I intend to show the same respect to all the patients that I encounter throughout my nursing career.

Elyse Ingle, BSN, RN

Finding Inspiration

I initially thought about the field of nursing because I knew it would provide a stable job with many opportunities. When I decided that I wanted to study nursing, I got strong oppositions from my family. Back in India, where I am from, nursing is not the highest or most acclaimed job. It's often looked down upon, even though times have changed and the profession is considered one of the most trusted. Skilled people still consider nursing to be a low-income service job. Most Indian parents want their kids to become a doctor, engineer, or lawyer. Yet, here I am. I chose nursing,

However, I can say one thing with confidence. Every time I go to work or clinical, as tired as I am and as much as I might say the night before I don't want to wake up, once I'm in a room taking care of a patient my attitude changes. Exactly how this mechanism works I still don't know. Is it the thank you after relieving a patient's pain? A smile from their family members when they know I'm taking great care of their loved one? Is it when I've had to reassure a patient as they fight in pain but look me in the eye with peace? I can't pin point any particular situation, but all of them, every single one of my patients, have impacted me. I believe that one has to find inspiration and motivation every day a patient doesn't thank you; when their family scrutinizes your every action; or when the patient screams to keep doing what they do every day. Sometimes you have to find inspiration even when your patient screams that you can't be their nurse even though you know you've given the best quality care

I love what I do, and I'm inspired and humbled every day to be given the chance to care for each and every one of my patients.

Feba Jacob, BSN, RN

A Mission Trip

The patient that really touched me as a student and made me realize that I chose the right profession was an Indian lady I met in Mexico while there with a student group. She came to a post-operative room from surgery. She had come to our clinic with her husband and one of her children from a far place. Her post-operative condition was severe. She was suffering pain from the side effects of antibiotics. She was enduring pain by clenching her teeth and shedding tears, and she tended to tolerate the pain without seeking help. I had to assess her pain level by observing her face. In addition, she couldn't understand Spanish because that was not her native language. I had to communicate with her through an interpreter or other family member who could translate her language to Spanish. It was hard to find a person who could translate each time. I tried to communicate with her by using gestures and face expressions. When she was suffering pain, I tried to give her emotional support with appropriate touch. Her family had stayed with her because they didn't have a place to stay. They willingly helped to take care of her. After a couple days, we could communicate even though we didn't have a common language. Unfortunately, we had to teach her husband low to care for her once home. He made a strenuous effort to learn, and we discharged them with the needed supplies. On the last day her little son came to me and gave me a hug with a nice smile. Before they left, she also came to me and gave me a hug and a kiss. If she had not gotten the surgery, she couldn't live for a long time. Even though we discharged her before she was in stable condition, it might be better than no surgery. However, I was very worried about her. I couldn't control my emotion and cried in front her. She took my hand and gave me a nice smile. Her husband showed me the supplies and gave me a smile with nodding. I have never forgotten their smiles. Their smile was greater than any words. I thought that nursing is a great job because we can be involved in people's lives and directly get their appreciation. In addition, we can work all over the world to save people.

Minami Kakuta, BSN, RN

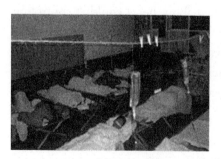 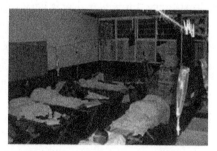

Views of the mission's post-surgical rooms

A Patient's Impact

During my first semester in nursing school, I had a patient that made a big impact on my life. She was a sweet woman in her 60's who was admitted for a broken hip. She could hardly walk or get out of bed. When I was assigned to her, she seemed somewhat hesitant to have me taking care of her at first. To gain her trust, I helped her with breakfast by cutting her pancakes and opening her milk carton while having a conversation about her and her family. Throughout the day when I was assessing her and administering her meds, she slowly opened up to me, cracking a joke once in a while and encouraging me on my skills.

Later that day, she asked me to give her a warm sponge bath in bed. While washing her back, she was telling me about her children and how they lovingly took care of her at home. She said that I reminded her of her children in a way because of my demeanor and personality. After I finished giving her a sponge bath, I dressed her and styled her hair. At the end, she gave me a great big smile and said, "Thank you so much for everything you did for me today. I really so appreciate it. I can really see that you care for your patients. You will be a great nurse in the future." I smiled back and replied, "You're welcome. Thank you for this great opportunity in taking care of you."

Till this very day, her words have kept me going. Every time I hear a patient say, "Thank you" or "I appreciate what you have done for me" or when a family member thanks me, it gives me the determination to continue to serve others and excel in being a nurse.

Rima Kanarch, BSN, RN

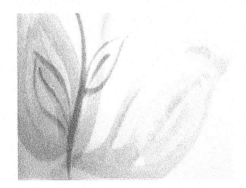

Unconditional Care

"So, Mr. W* is so uncooperative, he refused wound care, and honestly there is no hope for him if he's not willing to help himself," the night nurse complained as she finished up report to the daytime nurse and myself.

At that moment, I decided I would not let their prejudice of an individual I have never met, let alone cared for, cloud my judgment and compromise care. Minutes later after pulling medications, the RN and I entered Mr. W's room with a warm "good morning."

"Later I'm going to release the crackin," Mr. W replied, which the RN simply logged into the computer and ignored him.

"Oh really," I joked and started a conversation with him as I completed my assessment

I could tell just from the RN's reaction during hand-off and her interaction with him during medication administration that I would need to assume care over this patient for the day to learn his mannerisms and discover reasoning behind his non-compliance. An hour later I returned to his room to teach Mr. W how to change his dressing and check on his wound vac with the wound nurse. The wound care nurse tried to show him how to change his dressing on his abdomen and also how to empty his colostomy bag, but he was uninterested and discontent.

After the wound care nurse left I decided to stay in the room and work with him on using his incentive spirometer, get him up and walking, and try to get to know him in the process. Mr. W told me that he hadn't been so great to his family and that he wasn't too surprised that they hadn't come to visit since he'd been there or even during surgery. I didn't want to pry or pass judgment, but I learned that he had a drinking problem which was the cause of his necrotic intestine and need for colostomy.

Though Mr. W didn't cooperate at first, after he opened up to me and shared his story, I realized he was lonely and remorseful.

"Well, Mr. W, I'm leaving for the day, but I wish you the best of luck and thank you for letting me work with you today," I said at the end of my day.

"No, thank you, and you are going to be a real good nurse," Mr. W replied.

At that moment I felt relief, hopefulness, and gratitude for getting the opportunity to care for a kind individual who just needed human interaction and an ear to listen. My previous experiences that I was contemplating began to vanish, and I knew I had chosen the right path.

Chelsea Kirkwood, BSN, RN

Patient's initial was changed to protect patient confidentiality.

The Moments That Make Life Meaningful

When entering nursing school I wasn't quite sure what type of experiences I would encounter or what I would be able to get out of the profession. After experiencing this situation with a patient, I realized that what I do as a nurse impacts others and they can impact my life as well.

One day on my nursing unit there was a man that had Guillain-Barrre Syndrome and due to this disease he was unable to feed himself. Due to the fact that I was a nursing student, I had the chance and the time to help feed this man. He wasn't able to vocalize his wishes because he had a trach. Slowly and patiently I tried reading his lips, and I was able to feed him exactly what he wanted and to his liking. It was amazing to see the simply joy of this man to be able to finally eat food, after several weeks of being NPO and not able to swallow. This man was so kind to me and thankful for spending the time to help feed him. I told him that it was my pleasure and that it was not a problem because I could tell he felt that he was bothering me or taking away my time. I reassured him that I enjoyed helping him and he smiled. Later, I found out that it was his birthday that day, and it really affected me that this man was spending his birthday in a hospital bed. I will always remember this man and the image of him smiling at me as I helped him do what all of us take for granted: to eat. It made me realize that what I do as a nurse, to help others in their most vulnerable state, is the most rewarding thing that I could ever do with my life.

Sharon Kluger, BSN, RN

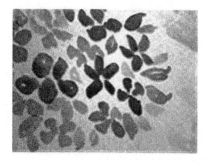

My First Patient

I will never forget my first patient. Given, it was my first day of clinical ever, I was terrified, nervous, and had no idea what to expect. I had never interacted with a patient before.

I took an extensive health history on a woman who was only in her mid-thirties and had a laundry list of chronic illnesses, tracheostomy, and was diagnosed with thyroid cancer. She was a former smoker of three packs a day for approximately twenty years. She also told me that she was a post illicit drug user, a single mom with a husband in jail, and her financial struggle was only one of her many problems at home. She said that her young boys were made fun of at school for having a mom that talked funny and had a hole in her neck. What worried her the most was the fact that her children might out live her one day. During our interview, she cried and asked me to hold her hand, stating that she would take it all back if she could go back in time. She now lives with emotional distress, depression, regret, and guilt for her past decisions that impacted her health and family so significantly.

This experience was eye opening for me. I realized not only how important it is to build a trusting relationship with a patient, but, more importantly, how precious life is and how many things people take for granted. That day I walked into that hospital room afraid of what to expect with nursing school and whether or not it was a good fit for me. That day I walked out feeling empowered knowing that nurses can, in fact, make differences in people's lives and this is exactly where I am supposed to be.

Katherine Knapp, BSN, RN

Experiences in the Pediatric Intensive Care Unit

At a very young age, Brian* was in a devastating car accident. Brian was found unconscious at the scene of the accident, was given CPR for two minutes, and was flown to the emergency department. Brian suffered a spinal cord injury at the C4-C5 level. Amazingly, Brian's cognition remained unaltered. After the accident Brian was placed on a ventilator, with a tracheotomy soon to follow. Since the damage occurred in the cervical spine, Brian lost sensation and function of all four extremities. One month after he arrived at the hospital, Brian became my patient.

The first day of Pediatric Clinical Rotation, after touring the hospital, I was dropped off at the pediatric intensive care unit for three hours, which was the unit I was assigned the following week of clinical. It was then that I met Brian and his primary nurse. Four days prior, Brian had become septic. He underwent an emergency procedure. Despite the frightening near-death experience, Brian's spirit lit up the room. His inflated tracheotomy cuff prevented Brian from speaking but that did not stop him from communicating. By shaking his head no and blinking both eyes for yes, Brian communicated with family members and caregivers.

Not only was Brian an adorable, bright-eyed young boy, he was able to teach his nurses a lesson in the strength of the human spirit. In the brief time that I spent on the PICU, Brian touched my heart and by the end of the day, I knew that I wanted to be a pediatric nurse.

Jessica Christensen Kruse, BSN, RN

*The patient's name was changed to protect patient confidentially.

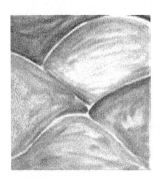

A Critically Ill Patient

It was the first week of my summer internship in the Intensive Care Unit (ICU), and my patient was a 20-something year old guy who had crashed his motorcycle several weeks before. I took care of him for three shifts, but I will never forget his name, his story, his family, or the impact it had on my development as a nurse. He had a traumatic brain injury, two broken arms, and assortment of scrapes and bruises, and was unresponsive. I was overwhelmed by all the equipment and tubes: ventilator, monitors, PEG tube, IV drips, and EVD. More unnerving, though, was the fact that none of my patients in previous clinicals had ever been unconscious, had brain injuries, or had such a poor, or at least unknown, quality of life prognosis. His parents were there during every visiting hour. It broke my heart to see them come in and talk to him and hold his hand, desperately looking for any glimmer or recognition in his blank stare. They were so sweet, and in so much pain.

I was struck by the realization that this broken person in the bed was utterly dependent on us for everything, and what an immense responsibility it is to care for such a patient. Although we could do little to repair his brain, every effort were did, such as bathing him, making him comfortable and presentable for his family, talking to his parents and being a listening ear, talking to him despite being unsure of his awareness, made a difference in this family's life. We were entrusted with the care of their beloved son, and to my surprise it was immensely rewarding to perform that care. I hope that as I graduate soon and begin practice as an RN, I can always preserve that sense of responsibility, and remember what an honor it is to take care of people in the most vulnerable and painful times of their lives. As a nurse, I can make a difference in the lives of my patients and their families, and I want to do that in the best way possible.

Nicole LaSalle, BSN, RN

A Patient Who Made A Difference

A patient that I have had that has really touched me would be one that I had on a surgical unit who just had a trach inserted. He was re-learning how to communicate and was really upset about everything that was going on in his life. He could no longer speak and had to talk to people through hand gestures and pen and paper. I could tell that it was frustrating trying to say something while not wanting to write down every little word. I took time to sit down with him and his wife and learn about their past and where they came from. They were from out of town and they were a little scared to be in a new hospital and new environment while going through such a rough time. They had no other family in the area so they were literally all alone. This man really opened up to me and explained how he was feeling at all times. He was going through a rough patch, but I sat down and took the time to understand him and talk him through his feelings. Every day he had his wife bring a huge bucket of candy and he always had little notes written on paper of things to tell me about when I returned the following week for clinical. He was in the unit for a long time and I got to know him on a more personal level than most patients. Every day I was there he told me how much he appreciated me and how, in little ways, I made an impact on his hospital stay. He made me feel welcome and was not afraid to ask for things he wanted/needed. I tried to make myself available to him at all times, and I felt he was in dire need of some attention. In the middle of nursing school he reminded me of why I joined nursing school and why I wanted to make a difference in people's lives for a living. He was an older gentleman and I almost looked to him, like a grandpa. I know in reality that I will not have this kind of time to sit down with patients, but while I'm in nursing school I wanted to learn from a patient's perspective. He actually taught me more than I expected, and I grew just from knowing him. He helped me learn different communication techniques and how to communicate through body language and eye contact. I will never forget this gentleman, and he has impacted my nursing career in more ways than he will ever know.

Lindsey Ledbetter, BSN, RN

A touching story

On the first week of acute course clinical rotation, I had the opportunity to take care of a gentleman from out of town who was staying with a family member at that time. At the end of the day, I went to the patient's room to say goodbye to him and his family. When I told them that I was leaving for post conference the patient said "But you are coming back later, right?" When I said "no" he immediately responded with "How about tomorrow?" It was a great feeling that a patient expressed a strong desire for me to come back to take care of him again. Furthermore, the patient's very elderly mother said "You did a great job taking care of my son. We need more people like you!" Hearing this from the patient's mother, who had been-a nurse for 35 years, was simply amazing and touching beyond description. All the tiredness melted away when I heard a comment like that. Right at that particular moment, I came to realize that I had chosen the right profession.

Eun Lee, BSN, RN

I Learned to Listen

In first semester, I cared for a young woman in her twenties. She was a beautiful girl with long dark hair and a pretty face. She had small children and was a single mother. She suffered from a disorder that caused her to need several surgeries including the one that she was recovering from during this hospital stay, which left her with a colostomy. She had been having difficulty with her body image stating concerns about how she would socialize, and even date, with the colostomy. She was frustrated by receiving differing and conflicting information about how to care for her stoma from various nurses and other healthcare professionals in the hospital. She told me of a horrifying experience in trying to change her colostomy bag and having it explode, making a mess everywhere while there was a provider in the room.

I related to this patient, as I am a woman about her age, and I have two small children. I could only imagine what she was going through in a world where looks are so important, and trying to deal with a condition that would probably be a put off to a young man. I felt for her.

Although I was only a first semester student who barely had any nursing skills besides how to take vitals, do an assessment and make a bed, the thing that I could do that I didn't need to learn in class, was to be a good listener. I listened to her frustrations and held her while she cried. I helped her into the shower and worked with a PCA to help her figure out a method of showering with the new stoma that worked for her. I thought a lot about her in the following weeks and I wanted to share a poem with her. The poem was called *Phenomenal Woman* by Maya Angelou. It's an uplifting poem that talks about the beauty, majesty and grace that all women possess. To me it was important for her not to feel as if she had been somehow damaged by her condition, that she was just as valuable and beautiful today as she was before the surgery. I hope that just being there for her, with a caring ear was in some way helpful to her on her journey. I don't think anyone had really done that during her stay. This experience helped me to realize that nursing is so much more than passing out medications and changing beds and physical assessments. It taught me that assessing the patients' emotional wellbeing is important as well. Also listening can sometimes be just as therapeutic as a pill.

Lucinda Lundy Zeinelabdin, BSN, RN

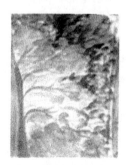

A Grateful Patient

While in nursing school, I worked as a Patient Care Assistant in a transplant intensive care unit. I was able to work alongside a nurse and help take care of a patient who eventually changed my view of nursing. The patient arrived on my unit in a critical state with more lines running through her than I had seen in my entire student nursing career. She was intubated, and the only noise in the room was that of my own footsteps as I proceeded to do my daily rounds of checking patients' rooms. As I was leaving, I noticed the patient had a wedding ring on. I instantly thought "Wow" looking at this lady in such a state. What if some day that was my wife or daughter; could I be able to handle seeing them in this condition? Over the next several days the family members arrived to see their relative for maybe the last time. What was even more heartbreaking was that the patient had several children, one who was currently in an ICU as well. Still every day I came into work surprised to see her still lying in bed. I couldn't believe that she was actually doing better. As days went to weeks and weeks to months, she did better. I could not have even imagined the day I would be able to sit there and have a conversation with this very grateful women. Not only was the patient grateful but the family was as well.

During her long stay in the ICU, I was able to observe and participate with the patient's health care. I could not help notice that the nurses were some of the most caring people that I have ever seen. I also saw firsthand how important nurses are to a patient's health. What makes a great nurse? Before this situation I would hesitate to tell you. Along with the nurse, the rest of the health care team was amazing. They all communicated well with each other and the family. Not once did a family member have to ask what is going on with my wife's care; what doctors are taking care of her; why haven't we seen a doctor today. The situation truly touched my heart and made me realize that I wanted to be just like those nurses.

Antonio Manocchio, BSN. RN

A Special Patient

My initial clinical experiences had allowed me to work with a variety of patients that had all impacted my education. Each patient had taught me a lot about the nursing field and allowed me to hone in on my technical skills. Especially in third semester, I had built more confidence and was given the freedom to practice more on my own under close supervision. The information we learned in class and had been tested on was starting to come full circle. As much as my patients allowed me to practice nursing skills, one of the most rewarding encounters with a patient reminded me to always remain true to myself.

A man that I had met during Adult I clinical had explained that he felt he was not receiving the best care. He explained that he felt his nurses and techs were giving him attitude and were not being attentive to his comfort needs. Although he was receiving the proper nursing care concerning medication and etc.; he still felt uncomfortable. He felt the nurses did not treat him with respect. Hearing his story of how the man felt he was treated, I felt appalled. No matter how good a nurse could be from his/her information, it is imperative to be sensitive to a patient's needs.

This just reaffirms my passion for nursing as I always try to treat others with extreme kindness and be there for them to the best of my abilities. I know that through nursing, I will be able to build personal relationships. I want to be able to make my patients feel comfortable to talk to me about their concerns. I have found it so rewarding to be able to nurse someone back to health, but most importantly, one must remain true to basic human instinct which is to treat others with kindness and respect. This behavior cannot be emulated through a textbook, and I feel it is a strong attribute I bring to the nursing field. This is one of the reasons I have chosen this profession and after this experience with this particular patient, I want to touch many lives and provide them with the best care possible.

Jesus Martinez. BSN, RN

A Pediatric Patient

One patient that really stands out to me was a baby I took care of in third semester pediatrics. He was eight months old and was recently diagnosed with a brain tumor. I immediately felt empathy for his parents who were standing over his crib crying. They told me how he hadn't been acting normal since his birth, but at the same time they seemed strong and hopeful that the doctors would do anything and everything to make their baby better. This baby made me realize why I wanted to be a nurse and how much healthcare professionals can make a difference in someone's life. The parents of the baby boy were just happy to talk to the doctors and nurses regarding their son. They also told me how safe they felt leaving him during the day while they went to work or tended to their five other children. I realized that nursing isn't always skills and knowledge, but it also involves being able to care and understand your patient's needs. I think that is why I want to be a nurse, at the end of the day I like to believe I can improve and impact someone's life.

Jackie Medintz, BSN, RN

A Patient Who Inspired Me

One of my most memorable patients was a young man in his teens who had been in a house fire. He was at a friend's house asleep at the time of the fire. He looked perfect on the outside, with no external burns and only a little edema; however, his throat and lungs were severely burned from inhaling all the hot smoke. He was on a ventilator, an ECG monitored his heart, and a drainage tube coming from his lungs was draining what looked like tar but was really all the dead burnt tissue. I learned that when someone is on a ventilator they also have to be paralyzed, but that does not mean that they cannot feel anything or hear you. Even though the patient looked completely unconscious my nurse explained to the patient that she had to put an NG tube down his throat so that he could get the nutrition he needed for his body to heal. She also prepared him that it would be painful due to the burns down his throat. As she slid the tube down, tears rolled down the sides of his face. I grabbed hold of his hand and spoke to him until she finished, attempting to distract and comfort him from the pain. His family was there by his side the whole time. You could see the fear in their eyes and they looked exhausted. It was then that I knew it was my duty to provide strength and comfort to not only my patient but the family as well. That was the day I put it all together and truly experienced what nursing is all about, combining both holistic nursing care with the use of best practice and knowledge. In that moment I knew, this is right where I needed to be

Karen Michalec, BSN, RN

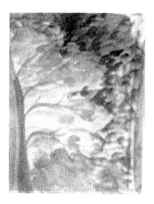

My "A Ha Moment"

I haven't always thought of myself as a nurse. There were many times during nursing school that I would second guess my decision to go into nursing. Several times throughout my time in nursing school, people would tell me that they think that I would be a great nurse and they'd wish me well. However, there was one person that stuck out for me and really helped me realize that I am doing what I have been called to do.

It happened one day when I was caring for an older gentleman whose health was deteriorating and was known for being "grumpy." After introducing myself, a few minutes of small talk ensued. He then asked me what brought me to nursing, and as I answered, he listed intently. Every time I walked into his room that day, his face would light up and he would start singing. At the end of the day, as I was saying my good buys, he reached out and kissed my hand. He told me that I would be a great nurse because if I could make a grumpy old man's day nice, I had what it takes to care for anyone.

Tanya Micheletti, BSN, RN

A Fun and Genuine Patient

I worked with Peggy* for her two days post-op after her second brain surgery. I went in at 6:45 am to introduce myself. She groggily replied with a friendly hello. She had a large bandage on the right side of her head, and I figured she would be sleeping that day. Later we got to talking, and it turned out she had her RN license. She was a character, and I enjoyed visiting her room during those two days. Many times she spoke highly of me and said I could be her nurse anytime the way I took care of her. She was extremely positive and upbeat despite the long road she had come. She had unexplained migraines for years and had been in the hospital many times for different surgeries, both exploratory and interventional. Peggy bounced back surprisingly quickly and was discharged the third day after all her surgeries. Her neurosurgeon kindly referred to her as his "mutant." Her medical challenges had not stopped her from living life to the fullest. She had many other careers besides nursing and had travelled the world.

We bonded those two days and by the end she gave me her number in case I ever needed any travel or nursing connections. She was only in her 40's, but she had done so much in her life and was the most fun and genuine person I have ever met. I will never forget Peggy. She was an inspiration to me both as the nurse and person I strive to be like every day.

Luka Micke, BSN, RN

Patient's name and identifying details have been changed to protect patient confidentiality.

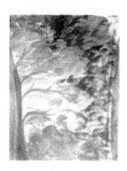

Angels

I walked into my patient's room during second semester thinking it would be just another clinical day. She was an older woman with many physical problems and a hard life. For a few hours, she remained tacit, not wanting to actively engage in conversation. I came and went about my business and most of the morning passed by uneventful. The doctors made their rounds and I entered my patient's room after catching bits and pieces of their discussion. There was my little lady in tears sitting quietly in her bed. I sat down and she started to talk. She wanted to go home, want to be well; she wanted a better life. I sat there listening to her heart-felt words and realized she needed someone who would listen. I stayed with her until lunch, and upon leaving her room was humbled by what came next. She asked me, "Are you an angel? God must have sent you to take care of me today. I asked Him for someone to help me and He sent you." Those words touched me deep inside and reaffirmed my decision to become a nurse. You know when you're in the right place if you can walk in a room a stranger and leave an angel.

Crisann (Dodgen) Moon, BSN, RN

A Wound Care Patient

I have had many experiences that have solidified for me why I chose nursing, and confirmed for me that I indeed made the right decision. One particular patient stands out in my mind as I reflect. Early in my nursing school career I had a patient who was suffering from a chronic wound which was infected and required packing. She was very nervous about how she was going to take care of her wound at home. She had no way to pay for her hospital stay, and she was being discharged before she really felt ready. I have to admit I was concerned for her to go home as well because her wound was on her coccyx and there was truly no way she could pack it and change the dressing on her own. She could not afford home care for someone to come and take care of her wound, and her daughter was overwhelmed by the task. I knew that if a solution was not found she would end up with a larger wound and back in the hospital. I worked to find resources for my patient to help her once she went home. I remember sharing with my instructor my concern and she too helped me to connect with social work and find a way to get the patient some form of home care. This situation and others much like it make me realize that I have been blessed with knowledge that the general population may not have, and it is my job to advocate for my patients and find solutions to problems that seem too complex for them to solve on their own. I was there for my patient that day. I listened compassionately to her concerns and did what I could to find her help.

Allison Moreno, BSN, RN

A Spanish Speaking Patient

Back in first semester of nursing school, I had a mid-fifties Hispanic lady whom had had a stroke and was receiving dialysis. On her chart, I had observed she was diagnosed as a demented patient whom was not compliant with her medications. Due to this massive hemorrhagic stroke, she was in a very detrimental condition. I picked her as my patient and was told speaking to her was very difficult to do because she mumbled. When I had heard report in the morning, it was noted she spoke nonsense and probably required to go to a psych ward. When I walked in to the room, I expected to her nonsense from this lady as I had been told earlier. I introduced myself and tried to carry a conversation with her. To my surprise I actually began understanding what she was saying. It wasn't so much that she mumbled nonsense; it was just that the stroke affected her speech. In addition, what sounded like gibberish was in fact Spanish she was speaking. I began asking her questions about her condition and although it was a bit difficult to understand, she did make sense. When one of the nurses was feeding her through her PEG tube, the patient began complaining that she was being fed too fast to which the nurse hadn't understood because she didn't speak Spanish. So I translated for her letting the nurse know that feeding her this fast made her extremely uncomfortable. Fortunately, the nurse slowed the feeding. Throughout the day I carried conversations with her and asked her about her life. She answered all of them and felt she was finally heard by someone. Holding this lady's hand made me see that nursing is indeed the career choice for me. I believe nursing is my vocation, my calling.

Rocio Neri, BSN, RN

My Inspiration

I got a chance to volunteer with the International Nurse's Students Association at a local festival in town. I had always wanted to offer my nursing services to the community and this opportunity was a perfect one. I thought it was going to be like any other screening experience but this one lady made the day for me. She was a lady in her sixties with no history of diabetes of hypertension. She was accompanied by her daughter who came to enjoy the festivities. I was assigned to offer patient education (the final station of the screening) at that time. When I looked at the patient's chart, I realized that her blood glucose was 34 and immediately knew that I had to intervene. My instincts "told" me to run to my instructor and the graduate student for advice or at least a go ahead to intervene, but they were away assisting at an emergency. So I immediately took charge, assessed her for signs of hypoglycemia (which were not apparent) and issued the lady a boxed apple juice, which was the only juice available, and asked her to rest for about 15 minutes before I checked her blood glucose again. Meanwhile I educated them on the symptoms of hypoglycemia together with other educational materials. I later checked her blood glucose which came up within the normal range. The lady and her daughter were very grateful for my help. The fact that I was able to identify a problem, assess the patient, intervene, evaluate and educate the patient was very rewarding. I got the chance to educate my colleagues on how to monitor for out of normal blood glucose ranges and the importance of reporting it promptly for the patient's safety. I believe this lady felt very well taken care of, and I was left very satisfied knowing that I was in the right profession to change lives and make people feel better than when I met them,

Winifred Ojowa, BSN, RN

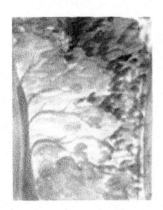

Inspiring Patient Experience

During my clinical experiences it was the patients that thanked me for my hard work, the ones that have a smile or joke for everyone that comes in, and the patients that remind me to keep things in perspective. One such patient, in spite of her physical disabilities and medical issues, could still find joy and happiness in life and then share that with everyone around her. Unfortunately, on a day I cared for this particular patient all the techs and I were kept occupied by the unforeseen issues and concerns of the other patients' requiring our immediate and undivided attention. Those patients kept me occupied for about an hour. Or course it was during that time this particular patient had an accident in the bathroom. The patient's family very calmly and politely requested housekeeping to clean the bathroom. Periodically when I passed the patient's room the family politely and very respectfully let me know housekeeping had yet to arrive. This patient and family never complained or got upset about the delay. I thanked them for their patience, cooperation, and understanding and assured them housekeeping had been notified and should be on their way. The family went to the extent of offering to clean the restroom themselves, if I could get them the supplies, because they could see how busy everyone was and were anxious to get it cleaned more for the roommate's comfort than their own. When I finally was able to stop by the room and check with the patient, they were extremely grateful and appreciative for the work I had done for them. Something that surprised and humbled me most was their concern for me in coping with that morning and apologized for adding to my work load. The patient and family thanked me profusely for the outstanding and conscientious care I had provided to the whole group and remarked on the kind of nurse I would be upon graduating. It is this type of patient and family that puts a smile on my face, a spark of happiness in my heart, and reaffirms my decision to pursue a career in nursing, even on my worst day.

Kristin Olsen, BSN, RN

A Young Soldier

I had the pleasure of working with a young soldier who fought for our country. When he was oversees he stepped on a land mine and lost both of his legs and had several more injuries. He was going through rehab, learning how to walk again and adjusting to his new life. You could tell that he was tired and emotionally drained from his last month's journey. Nevertheless, he stayed positive, and his will to fight and succeed did not diminish. His wife was always by his side and they were talking about children and future plans.

This patient showed me that I am in the right profession because by helping I was able to make a difference. I was providing teaching and support to him and his wife emotionally by listening. I was also able to see that no matter what life throws at you, you are capable of recovery with proper help and love.

Going through the clinical experiences I realized that every single patient I had touched me and made me realize that I enjoy helping people and love seeing the outcome. Seeing people smile, feel comfortable and good the day I care for them makes me feel satisfied and fulfills me.

Kristina Omisola, BSN, RN

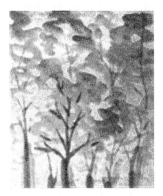

A Little Boy

The one patient that moved me in many ways was a little boy who was in a motor vehicle accident. His mother had strapped him in to his car seat, but the car seat had not been strapped into the car properly. His mother, the mother's boyfriend, his aunt, and the little boy were all in the same car when they were in the accident. The boyfriend was killed, the mother was seriously injured, the aunt was injured as well, and the little boy and the car seat were thrown like a missile out of the car. The little boy ended up with a broken neck. He was paralyzed from the neck down, was on a ventilator, and was being fed through a G-tube. He had been life-flighted to this hospital, while his mother was recovering in a hospital several hours away. All he could do was lay there and watch a TV that the nurses had placed in front of him. His whole world had changed in a split second and nobody that he was familiar with was at his bedside. He could not make any sounds but he would pucker up his lips like he was crying, and he had tears in his eyes. He was probably wondering where his mother was. I read to him, bathed him, stroked his head and hair since that is the only place he still had feelings, and spoke lovingly to him. It was very difficult as I would start choking up while watching this poor baby lay there so helpless. He spoke only Spanish, so I tried to say as many Spanish words as I could remember. The words, "Whatsoever you do to the least of my brothers, you do unto me" came of my mind. This was Jesus in disguise. I often wonder how this little boy is doing, and when I think of him I am so thankful for the many blessings in my life. It was a great feeling and privilege to be able to tend to this baby boy, and I knew that day that I had chosen the right career.

Alaina Paglia, BSN, RN

Significant Patient

It was another busy day on the medical-surgical unit, and I was completing morning assessments on my patients. I had visited the first two and was making my way into the last patient's room. When I told her hello, she instantaneously clicked and I knew she felt comfortable with me. Throughout the day, I visited with her and her family and we talked about her slight progress, the horrific lunch she was supposed to eat, and my education. After lunchtime she opted to take a shower because she said she felt comfortable with me assisting her. She had been diagnosed with lung cancer one year ago, and it had recently metastasized to her brain. She confided in me that she didn't want to get her hair wet because it had recently started to grow back in the smallest patches. When it was time for me to leave the unit, she praised me for my nursing skills and told me I would be the best nurse because I knew the importance of caring for my patients.

The next day she was not on the unit and I coincidently ran into her sister in the hospital elevator. She was so excited to see me and said her sister had been asking for me every time a healthcare member came into the room. She said her health had dramatically declined and she would truly appreciate it if I stopped by to see her. The next week, I took the time after clinical to stop by and see how she was doing. When I stepped into her room, I couldn't even recognize her because of how thin and frail she had become. She smiled at me but didn't have the strength to speak. I kindly held her hand and told her I wanted to check on her and told her to get some rest. Before leaving her room, her sister approached me and told me the doctor said she would pass away at any moment. As she was talking to me she began to cry and for the first time, I didn't know what to say. I hugged her and fought the lump in my throat and told her to be strong for her sister. She wiped her tears away and told me that I really impacted her sister's life and she truly appreciated the tender care I gave to her in her expected last days.

That day I walked away from the hospital and felt a sense of peace in my heart. The nurses on this particular unit were not the most welcoming or friendly to me, which made me feel inadequate. But after this, I knew with 100% certainty that I had chosen the right profession and, most importantly, for the right reason.

Krystal Perez, BSN, RN

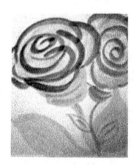

My Labor and Delivery Patient

I left the Air Force and headed for nursing school because I truly felt God was calling me to be a nurse. After seeing the devastation of Hurricane Katrina, I knew that I wanted to be in the position to help the next time there was a natural disaster or terrorist attack. On my first day of school I was completely preoccupied with the assignments I would have to write, clinical hours I would have to complete, and projects I would have to endure. I was completely distracted with all of my thoughts on what I would have to do to complete nursing school that it didn't even dawn on me that I was about to journey through such an incredible experience and was about to meet some amazing and wonderful people along the way.

One patient in particular confirmed my desire and decision to become a nurse. In my labor and delivery rotation, I met a 19 year old who was about to give birth to her first child. I helped her push for 3 hours and held her hand as she endured the contractions. I watched her cry and laugh, and I got to be a part of one of the most important days of her life. I held her hand when the doctor informed her that she would have to have a C-section, and at the end of the procedure, she told me that I kept her focused and she was thankful I was by her side. Those words to me meant more than any A on a test. I realized that the relationship between a patient and a nurse is so unique and special and I look forward to many wonderful years as a nurse.

Kelleah Pitts, BSN, RN

Answers

The reason I chose to become a nurse is because I love being able to offer comfort to people in their time of need or pain.

I had one patient in particular who really instilled in me the belief that I made the perfect choice when deciding on this career choice. Let's call him "Dan*." Dan had been in and out of the hospital and to multiple doctors, many times within the previous three months before I met him. He was brought into the unit I was working on after being admitted through the Emergency Department for shortness of breath and a persistent, dry cough that had been plaguing him for three months which became so severe that he would almost pass out from lack of oxygen during coughing fits

Once admitted onto my floor I had a chance to meet him and his wife. They were a newly married couple in their late 40's, both with children from previous marriages. They were very devout in their Christian beliefs and kept praying for answers. They had such positive attitudes throughout the entire time I saw them, and they were constantly laughing and saying how much they loved each other. It was very easy to see how genuine the love was between them.

Throughout the first day, Dan was taken for biopsies and chest and abdomen scans. Once the results came back the doctor came to the floor to give Dan and his wife the answers that they were desperately seeking about Dan's health. The doctor proceeded to explain some things and it came down to a diagnosis of inoperable lung cancer that had already spread to his liver and pancreas. The family was clearly upset so when the doctor left I offered to talk to them and offered empathy with the news they had received. It was very hard to sit with them and see the emotional strain it caused on their positive outlook. But even after all the bad news; Dan and his wife were thankful that their prayers had been answered about Dan's health.

I was glad to be able to be there and share the moment with Dan and his wife and offer what I could to them. I felt that just being able to do small things like hold his hand when he became upset and hug his wife when she needed a hug was wonderful. At the time my day was ending on the floor I went in to tell them goodbye and tell them how fortunate I was to be able to work with them that day. They were very sweet and told me what a great job I did, and that they really appreciated the time I spent talking with them. At the moment I walked out of his room, I was grateful that I was able to offer them empathy and compassion in their time of need and that choosing to be a nurse allowed me to do that.

Jennifer Polasek, BSN, RN

*Patient's name and exact situation was changed to protect patient confidentiality.

An Angry Patient

The one particular patient made me realize why I chose the right profession. My patient was admitted to the hospital for several diagnoses. He was a paraplegic due to a motor vehicle accident, and he had a history of broken bones. He was frustrated and expressed anger towards the world. He also lacked family support.

The day of my care, the patient expressed his anger towards the staff of the hospital. He verbalized things that shouldn't be publicly repeated. This patient was full of anger, frustration and hatred of the staff, and he felt his needs were not met. He expressed the lack of care from the staff and the lack of understanding of his illness. As a student taking care of the patient I was obligated, but not forced, to care for all the unnecessary things the patient articulated. Though I did provide the patient with care to the best of my ability, I did the things that the patent asked me to do and also provided him with emotional support. The patient really appreciated the services I had given him. I listened to his concerns and questions, and especially paid extra attention to his needs and wants. The patient was so grateful, and he told me that I was going to be a great nurse. It made me realize how important I was to his care.

Reynaldo Powao, BSN, RN

Fluff Is Good Medicine

It was in the place that I least expected when I finally got the confirmation I was looking for. I was debating the area of nursing to specialize in, even more, if nursing was right for me. I liked anatomy, physiology, and pharmacology, but the social aspect of nursing? Therapeutic conversation, patient family interactions. Fluff. I did not have the best attitude for the start of the semester, which included pediatrics and obstetrics. I considered this "girly stuff". I did not want to deal with children and had no interest in distraction techniques and developmental milestones, until I met him.

A typical start to any clinical day, buzzing on coffee in hopes it would get me through the shift. I picked up my assignment which included facial trauma, bloody wounds, and lack of family involvement. This was my kind of patient. When I walked into my patient's room, I was immediately struck by his demeanor: quiet, obedient, tough but sad. He showed his colors by gritting and bearing the excruciating pain of his dressing change without shedding as much as a tear. He never complained, never asked questions, and always took his medicine. Do they make kids like that anymore? The more I interacted and chatted with him, the more my shell began to soften and the more he cheered up. I learned that the family only had one car which the dad used for work which is why they had trouble getting to the hospital. However, they soon arrived with all the siblings in hand, and I was quickly booted out of the room.

I knew nursing was the career for me after that day. Although I still maintain that I will never go into pediatrics, I am so grateful for that experience and the opportunity to touch that little boy's life by providing my presence, although it was really he that touched me. Working with this boy reminded me that patients are human and humans need more than just interventions requiring skill. Holistic nursing is what makes patients better. I realized that the social aspect of nursing is not just fluff, it is good medicine.

Analisa Ramos, BSN, RN

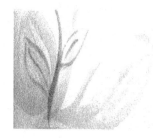

A Touching Patient

Sometimes the simplest things can make you happy. As I took care of a patient one clinical day, I did my assessment, gave him his medications, and all other things concerning his care as a nurse. About midway through the morning, he asked me why he had to have an IV line when he was not receiving any treatment by IV. I was happy to explain to him that if an emergency would happen and we needed to give him medication quickly, he already had an IV line available for quick and efficient access. As the patient, he was extremely grateful to know why he had an IV line. As a nurse it is something very simple to know, but he did not know. It really touched me to be able to give him something so simple as an explanation

Alicia Richesin, BSN, RN

A Little Girl in PICU

During my second semester of school, I had the honor to take care of a two year old precious little girl in the Pediatric Intensive Care Unit (PICU). She had been there several days prior to me taking care of her. She was there because he had been in a car accident with her mother and received extensive injuries. She had major spinal cord injuries, which resulted in her being a quadriplegic, although she was able to move her left arm, so I am not sure what that would be called. The reason why this case in particular touched me so much was because these injuries were somewhat preventable and resulted as a knowledge deficit in the mother. When the accident occurred, the child was sitting in a booster seat in the back seat. The seat belt is what caused the injuries to her spinal cord, almost snapping it into pieces. The mother said she thought it was ok to put her daughter in the booster seat, being she was big for her age (tall). All she needed was education about what is the proper equipment to use for her two year old, and this really could have been prevented. As nurses we are the last to see the patients and we need to make sure we educate them and allow them to feel comfortable to ask questions before leaving the hospital. A lot of times accidents happen due to lack of knowledge. What touched me most about this case was how strong the patient was. She was a happy and playful child that loved for someone to read her books. She was content with me telling her stories and reading her books. What stood out to me though, was that she would not let anyone touch her left arm, which was the only part of her body she could move. I believe it was more of being able to have some control over what was going on. It's very difficult to have to depend on people to do everything for you.

Takesha Roberson, BSN, RN

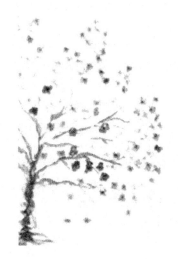

Nursing Experience

In my experience in the medical field, I have found that nursing is a career that must come from the heart. I would describe it as a natural aura that you can spot in any person. One case that accentuated my "aura" in nursing took place in the ICU. Upon walking onto the floor, I heard banging of side rails and feet slamming against the bed. The nursing staff eventually calmed this gentleman down. However, this patient continued to bang on his rails and yell at staff when they tried to help him. One time, while helping his nurse, I walked out of the room with a thank you from my nurse and _____ from the patient. One of the other nurses who had heard him stated "You shouldn't let him talk to you like that." With the situation in mind I had taken what the nurse said with a grain of salt. The patient had restraints on for getting aggressive with staff and had just been extubated the previous night, so he was already traumatized. Throughout the shift, he terrorized the staff with demands and constant banging of the bed rails.

The next week I returned to the hospital for another shift. I received report and walked onto the floor looking for my patient. Upon entering the room I noticed a young man gasping for air through an oxygen mask. His torso hunched as he sat on the bed staring at the floor. I put my hand on one shoulder, looked the patient in the eyes, and couldn't believe that this docile person was the same patient who was stressing the staff from last week.

During that shift, I received notice that he was placed on comfort care, meaning he would eventually die. Throughout the rest of my time, I helped the patient barely keep the oxygen mask on and treated him with the best care possible. He deserved the best even after what he had done to the staff and myself. I felt empathy for this patient. I couldn't help but think how horrible it would feel to die young and alone.

From ICU to Hospice nurse, I knew that I would treat any patient with the utmost respect. It's important to understand that we never truly know what these patients go through. Their lives are never only the complaints of your coworkers or what is in the charts. You need to take a moment to dive deep within your values and think about how you would want to be treated. This is why my heart is set on nursing and my aura continues to shine brighter and brighter each patient I touch.

Ryan Robisheaux, BSN, RN

Patient Who Touched Me As A Student

Being a fourth semester nursing student I can proudly say that I have had many wonderful experiences in every clinical setting. I also have had many positive encounters with patients and their families, nursing staffs, physicians, and my colleagues. During clinical I try to make the most of every opportunity given to me and continue to seek for high acuity patients to utilize my critical thinking in all aspects of care. To say the least, one morning I was placed in an intensive care unit and was assigned to a patient whom was well known by many. This particular patient had an effect on me the first minute I introduced myself. Being in the patient's position, one can assume a high level of frustration and possible hopelessness due to a past history of critical conditions. Throughout the day I was able to build a comfortable environment with the patient and family. Considering the patient's condition, anytime I would attempt to document or collaboratively discuss information with staff, my patient would look at me and wave with a smile. During nursing care and performing various skills, every so often the patient would shake my hand and inform me how appreciative he was of the care provided. On break I ran into a family member and she stated, "Thank you so much for all you have done. You are really doing an amazing job. I really appreciate it." Positive reinforcement and patient showing happy expressions always makes for a good day as a nurse.

Emil Sakhel, BSN. RN

My Patient Inspired Me

A patient I took care of in my second semester of nursing school inspired me in a way I didn't think was possible being simply a "nursing student". There was an elderly lady I was taking care of who was in the hospital for a persistent cough. While I was taking care of her, the doctor had given her the news that she had malignant cancer that had spread to her lungs and she had about six months to live. I had never been comfortable with the thought of death, and I felt I was in nursing school to help people live comfortably. For some reason the death of patients hadn't really occurred to me until this day. I thought I would be of very little use of this patient because all I had to do is give her a couple of pain pills and check her vital signs. Well, when I walked in to the patient's room she was crying. When I asked if there was something I could do for her it was like a flood gate of thoughts and words came towards me. I listened to her and she told me about her kids and how she was afraid to tell them about her impending death, about how some friends and family were coming and she didn't want them to see her "sick looking". When she was done talking about fifteen minutes later I had no magical words to make anything better or help her so I asked her if she wanted me to help her get dressed and put some makeup on so when her family came to see her she would not look "sick". To my surprise she was thrilled. At the end of the shift she thanked me over and over again, because I had listened to her and helped her during this difficult time. It was surprising to me because I didn't think I had done anything. I hadn't made her better, hadn't healed her in anyway. That is when it occurred to me. Nursing isn't just about making patients better; it's also about being comfortable with life and death, and treating not only the physical illness but also the emotional and frightened patient. It can be from simply listening when necessary

Melodie Saldivar, BSN, RN

My "A HA" Moment

I have always heard of people in nursing school having their "a ha moment." When I had my moment, it hit me so suddenly that when I started discussing it with my clinical instructor I found myself so overwhelmed at the love I had for my floor that I started crying. That day started as normally as possible at 5:30 am, I practiced my daily routine of getting into my scrubs and heading to the hospital just as I always had. When I was assigned to the Hematology/Oncology floor, I felt a pit in my stomach growing from the mixture of fear of not being able to control my emotions, and joy that I got to work in pediatrics. I made my way to the floor through the big double doors and was immediately greeted with friendly smiles and words of encouragement. I took a deep breath and tried to prepare myself for my day on the oncology unit. As soon as I walked into my first patient's room, my heart melted when I encountered the cutest little boy with superman pajamas and a Monsters, Inc. blanket. I walked over to say hello and began my assessment on him. I started my routine of taking his vital signs, and I noticed that he kept looking at me as if he was waiting for me to say something. His mother started giggling, and said that he had just learned to count and the other nurses would count with him while taking blood pressure. I immediately complied, as we giggled together while counting out loud to 10 as if it was the most exciting thing we would ever do. He was so proud of himself, puffing up his chest and pointing to the big "S" on his Superman pajamas. This little boy, although sick with cancer, had the most amazing outlook on life and looked forward to counting to 10 with his nurse as though it were Christmas morning. He continued to amaze me throughout the day, being such a brave boy while getting blood transfusions and taking his medications, which I knew did not taste very good. I found myself watching the clock and waiting until I got to go back into his room, so we could count to 10 together. I had a moment that day that took my breath away and left me dumbfounded when I realized that my little patient sitting in the hospital with cancer, had left me with a smile on my face that I could not get rid of. I was lucky enough to go visit him again the next day, and I caught him right before he was being discharged. He had gotten a new backpack to pack up all of his tiny clothes, and again, he was the happiest little boy I'd ever seen. As I said goodbye to my amazing little patient, he started walking away, his backpack hitting his heels and covering his entire body so that it looked as though a backpack was walking on its own. That picture, my "a ha moment," will always be burned into my brain as one of the most special times of my life.

Martita Sheesley, BSN, RN

Babies Depend on Nurses

The reason why I want to become a nurse is because I like to help others, especially those in need. I've been through four semesters of clinical and out of all the patients that I've taken care of newborns are the ones that have inspired me the most and made me realize I've chosen the right career. The first newborn that I took care of was during my OB rotation during second semester. This baby was premature and born to an incarcerated drug user. I will never forget how fragile this baby looked, how he jittered when touched and the sound of his high-pitched cry. Then, third semester, on my pediatric rotation, I got to work in the Neonatal Intensive Care Unit (NICU). There I took care of newborns abused by their parents and newborns with complex medical issues.

One thing that always stood out the most to me was how strong and resilient newborns are, even when the environment around them is so hostile. Babies are completely helpless when they are born, so in order to survive they depend on caring and competent parents. When you don't have reliable parents the chance of survival for these babies completely drops, so in my opinion that's where the role of nursing is very important. These babies now depend on nurses like me to make sure proper care is delivered. They depend on the information taught by the nurses to their parents and on the referrals to appropriate agencies that can help. Their resilience and knowing that their life many times depends on good nurses is what inspired me and made me realize that I'm in the right profession.

Keyster Silva, BSN, RN

The Patient That Changed My World

I was the first day of my pediatric clinical rotation. I had no idea what to expect or even how I was going to make it through the day. The thought of having to walk into a suffering child's room broke my heart and made me question all my beliefs about God. I slowly entered the elevator, pressed the floor number, and watched the doors close. I was telling myself that I have to be strong, because this child needs me. Finally, the elevator doors opened and I proceeded to my patient's unit. When I came to my patient's room, I caught myself having a hard time entering the room. I stood outside the room looking through the glass door wondering how much pain he was in, what his life could possibly be like living this way, and why did God do this to him. Finally, I forced myself to enter his room. He was lying on his back holding his Spiderman pillow while watching cartoons on the television. He noticed that I came in, and he turned my way to say hello. I could not believe how clear and strong he was talking on a ventilator. I told him hello and introduced myself. He was pleased to meet me and stated that he was excited to talk to someone new. I could not agree with him more. I was looking forward to getting to know him and understanding what his life was like. However, even though I was excited, I guess he noticed that I was nervous. He told me that there was no reason to be nervous. He was born with this condition and there was nothing we could do about it. He then proceeded to show me how to suction his tracheostomy, how he liked his pillows, and he explained his condition to me. I could not believe how much he knew, how emotionally strong he was, and how open he was about his condition. After he saw that my nervousness was settling down, he began to tell me about his life. He told me how he likes to play hide and go seek in his wheelchair and how he likes to spend time with his friends. He said that his favorite thing to do was to drive bumper boats. He stated that he loved life, and he would not wish to be anyone else because God made him that way. I could not believe what I was hearing. This child loved life more than anyone else that I have ever known. I was completely intrigued and inspired by him. He has so much life in him and so much to offer life. Towards the end of our conversation, the child's grandma came in the room. She asked him how he felt. He stated that he was in a lot of pain but that did not matter. He told his grandma to come sit down by him because he wanted to give her a birthday hug. At that moment, I knew I was in the right profession. I knew that God sent me to Earth to take care of sick children, because sick children will teach me more about life than life could teach me itself. By the end of the day, I no longer questioned God and truly understood the reason why sick children exist in this world. Before I left for the day, the child called me over and thanked me for listening to him. He told me that this was one of the best days he has ever had in the hospital - because of me. Who could ask for more?

Erika Sirchia, BSN, RN

Patient Who Touched Me as a Student

I had the opportunity during a clinical to care for a male in his sixties who was admitted with complications from severe type II diabetes. He had been in poor health for many years and had a long history of complications of type II diabetes and hypertension. During this visit to the hospital his left leg had been amputated at the hip.

During report my nurse told me that patient had been severely depressed and no one had been to visit him during this hospital stay. She asked that I spend some time with him and see if he would like to talk. I agreed to do so and went to introduce myself to the patient. To my surprise we hit it off quite quickly, and we spent several hours that morning talking.

He had no family as his wife had died 2 years earlier and they had not had any children. Many of his friends had died and he was in need of someone to talk to. We spent several hours talking about his life in this area and his career as a locksmith. Since his retirement and the death of his wife he had been very lonely, and due to his poor health, he was forced to spend most of his time alone in his small house. He welcomed the chance to talk to someone that morning, and I really enjoyed spending time with him. Since then I have often wondered whatever became of him.

Rodney Smith, BSN, RN

Why Nursing Is For Me

To understand the reason why nursing is the ideal profession for me, one must first know what drew me into the field. Shortly after graduating from high school, I was involved in a motor vehicle collision. I spent several weeks recovering from injuries acquired in the accident, including head injury/trauma. Once I improved in my mental status. I noticed the care that was being provided by nurses to me. After being released from the hospital, I began to realize how much the nurses had impacted my life. While I was recuperating from injuries that had me at the lowest part of my life, nurses were there to provide care and to help me realize how lucky I was to survive. They provided me with the optimism that I needed to help me look past my injuries and see the opportunities I had ahead of me. I decided to choose the profession of nursing to impact the lives of people in need, just like what was done to me.

Recently, I had a patient that reminded me of the incident I was involved in. The patient was also involved in a motor vehicle collision in which he received a head trauma. Although the patient couldn't see due to being sedated, I provided nursing care to the best of my ability throughout the day. I had the opportunity to converse with the family as they shared with me how grateful they were to have the nurse and I provide care for the patient. The expressed how previously they didn't have a good experience with another nurse. For the remainder of the day the sole reason why I chose the profession of nursing kept reiterating in my head. That reasons is impacting the lives of patients and their families in a positive manner.

Eli Solis. BSN, RN

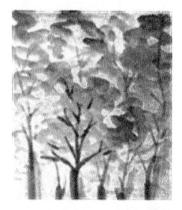

One Patient Vividly Remembered

I remember one patient vividly from my third semester of nursing school, and because of her, I know I chose the right profession. I showed up that morning and was assigned to a nurse just like every other morning. After reading all of the charts and listening to report, I chose Elaine* as my patient. It wasn't anything cool that a student would usually choose, but she spoke English and wasn't on a one to one [watch] like the other two, which was a great choice for me.

I went into her room and introduced myself to her like I would every other patient. She smiled up at me and said, "Good morning" even though I knew from her chart that wasn't the case. Elaine had a terrible abdominal obstruction and was in a lot of pain. They had already attempted to do a colonoscopy to determine the obstruction but the scope would not advance. They were still running tests on her and had not diagnosed the problem. At the end of the day, the physician informed her that they would be doing exploratory surgery the next morning to visualize the issue. Being the nursing student that I was, I was excited because I was going to get to see the procedure.

The next morning when I arrived, they were preparing her for transport. After they prepped her, they wheeled her down to pre-op where she waited. While in the room, her husband stepped out and she broke down. She started crying and expressed concern about the surgery and the possible outcome of a mass being the obstruction. I sat with her until she felt some peace of mind. After she finished crying, she thanked me for being with her and told me I was going to be a great nurse one day. I realized that nursing is not about skills or performing cool tasks. It is about the patient and creating that trust. That is the point I realized I had chosen the right profession.

Meaghan Stefanic, BSN, RN

*The patient's name was changed to protect patient confidentially.

A Special Child

During my pediatrics clinical I had to change my elementary school days and location due to scheduling conflicts. On my first day in the nurse's office I met a little boy names Dante*. He wasn't sick. He really just wanted to hang out and get some help with his math work. While we were chatting, I noticed he had a congenital ear deformity called microtia. The external ear never formed; there was a nub in its place. I found out from Dante and the nurse that his father and grandmother had taken him to several doctors, some as far away as California for treatment. No one would help him. They said he needed to wait 4-5 more years. As a surgical tech I have assisted on microtia reconstructions. It is divided into four separate procedures over a matter of months. A local doc is world renowned as a specialist in this treatment. I visited his website and was able to print information about the doctor and procedure in Spanish. Dad and Grandma weren't fluent in English. I gave the packet I created to Dante. He returned to school the next day and told me he had an appointment with the doctor soon. The school nurse exchanged email addresses with me so I could stay up to date on his progress. My semester became quite hectic and I never emailed her to follow up. Due to school, I was hardly ever at work. I happened to work one day in August and saw the surgeon to whom I referred Dante. I mentioned Dante to him and he knew exactly whom I meant. He told me that Dante had already had surgery and was doing wonderful. Without nursing I would never have met Dante. Knowing that

I made a difference in one child's life supports my decision to pursue a career that promotes beneficence and empathy.

Kristi Stuckey, BSN, RN

The patient's name was changed to protect patient confidentially.

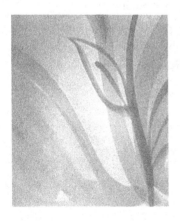

A Patient That Touched Me

I have had many patients during my time at nursing school. Some are more memorable for one reason or another, but one I will never forget.

I followed my nurse on her rounds as we went to the patients' rooms. The nurse told me she suspected one female patient was just a drug seeker. I noticed that the nurse was not very nice to her, and this patient was very sullen and lethargic every time we went into her room.

Later in the afternoon, I had extra time, so I went back in to check on this patient by myself. She still seemed distant and uninterested in talking, but I gently continued to talk with her in an empathetic and therapeutic manner. I asked her about what brought her here and her family, and I asked her about her feelings about her illness. She seemed to slowly see that I was interested in her and her story. She talked about her anxiety and issues at home that were brought on by her chronic illness state. I noticed that as we talked she became more engaged and came out of her shell. I couldn't believe that this was the same person we saw all morning long. Now she was finally smiling. She listened to me attentively when I suggested alternative avenues for dealing with her anxiety. I also taught her how to do some relaxation breathing exercises which we did together.

When it was time for me to go she smiled at me and intently told me that I would make a good nurse someday. I was in my first semester of nursing school, and I didn't feel like I was of much value to anyone at this point so I wasn't expecting any comment like this. It really touched me and made me happy that I brought a little relief to someone's life

I felt bad that the nurse was being pre-judgmental and had just written off the patient. No wonder the patient was so sullen. I am glad I chose to ignore the nurse's position and tried to treat the patient like a human instead.

Chris Sylvester, BSN, RN

My Niche

I spent my time as a nursing student constantly wondering where my niche will be following graduation. I constantly tried to meld myself into each environment – whether geriatrics, pediatrics, obstetrics, psych-mental health, acute, or medical-surgical – because nursing students are to have a general perspective of all the major specialties in order to provide adequate basic holistic care.

It wasn't until I chose oncology for my nursing elective that I was exposed to a setting that piqued my interest. I had a basic understanding of the theory behind and involved with cancer and its therapy from my course on management of chronic illnesses, but I was rarely exposed to the experience of this patient population. My clinical rotation was at a local cancer treatment facility. The patient population I was exposed to varied in types of cancers, ages of patients, previous treatment experiences of patients, and reasons of how and why the patient chose to have treatment at this facility.

The one patient that inspired me and helped me realize that I chose the right profession in nursing was the one patient I couldn't communicate with in English – this patient was middle-aged female who spoke only Spanish (a language I only had basic knowledge in speaking and comprehending). She had already gone through several conservative therapy sessions before this research faculty found her to be a good candidate for a study on an experimental drug. I had encounters with her during the early stages of the research paperwork –filing documentation for therapy—to the first series of her treatment. I spent several clinical days speaking in broken (and most likely incorrect, word use) of the Spanish language, but the language barrier was hardly a barrier at all. She responded back in a good-natured form, not annoyed at my attempts. There were moments when physicians assumed that I could act as a translator based on the therapeutic environment my patient and I had developed.

I didn't do a lot of hands-on skills and I didn't see immediate effects of my general presence, which would typically alarm me in my other clinical rotations. On a medical-surgical floor or in an ICU setting I needed to have interventions and outcomes. With my oncology patient, I was assured by no more than the environment that I could progress from a professional nursing student to a professional registered nurse.

Josephine Taele, BSN, RN

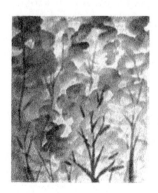

A Little Brother

Starting as a new nurse you never know in what way you will impact a patient or how a patient can so easily impact a new nurse. While working in the Pediatric Intensive Care Unit with a young child who had been recently diagnosed with a severe brain tumor, I was the student nurse who was so easily impacted by a patient. The young girl was extremely close to her little brother and just wanted so bad to make him happy while they spent time together. As I watched, she played with him and held him while she lay in pain and exhausted in her hospital bed. She was in such peace with him being around her, but it was soon time for him to head back home. I walked into the room and asked the young boy if he would help me do my assessment on his sister. He got to listen to her heart; he got to look into her eyes and to touch her face during a neuro assessment. He was allowed to take care of his sister just as she always took care of him. As their mother saw this, she thanked me and was so grateful for what I had done. To me though, I had done so little; let him use the flash light; let him use the stethoscope, nothing grandiose. Through the mother, the patient, and the brother, they taught me that the smallest gestures make the greatest impact, while hearing how appreciative and thankful they were. That small gesture helped me to realize what nursing is really all about.

Sara Talley, BSN, RN

A Patient Who Helped Me Realize I Chose the Right Career

Every patient I care for touches my heart in some way, but there is one that I won't ever forget. On my very first day of clinical in my first semester of nursing school I was assigned to a patient on a rehab floor. My patient was a woman in her 40's who had recently become paralyzed from the waist down after contracting spinal meningitis. I walked into her hospital room in the morning with my instructor, unsure of what to expect. I was surprised to find a very positive woman, determined to learn to work through her new disabilities and get back to her life and family. As I worked with her throughout the day, I felt humbled and privileged to have a complete stranger telling me about such personal thoughts and aspects of her life in such an open and trusting manner. I also realized that being able to establish a trusting working relationship with a patient was an essential skill, especially in that setting. The fact that I was terrible at reading a manual blood pressure was insignificant at that point. Getting confirmation on the very first day of clinical that I could be a caring nurse, and I loved doing it, has gotten me through the rough moments in nursing school.

Meghan N, Teran, BSN, RN

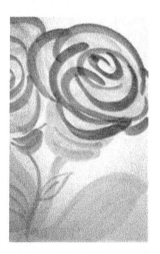

My Most Memorable Patient

There have been many different occasions where I have been able to step back and realize how much I love nursing and look forward to a future in it. However, there is one specific patient who comes to mind anytime someone asks me about my favorite/most interesting/most heart-wrenching experience. She was in her early twenties and was ten weeks pregnant with her first child. She had come to the Intensive Care Unit in code status due to septic shock. This patient was, by far, the sickest I had ever taken care of, so of course, I was instantly scared.

Her condition continued to worsen, and she ended up aborting the fetus while I was caring for her. I will never forget walking into the room with the mother and patient crying, then looking between her legs and seeing the little baby boy lying in the sheets. He was about the size of the palm of your hand. His hands, feet and facial features were all fully formed, and his umbilical cord was still attached. She and her family were devastated, yet never showed defeat.

It was never the patient's diagnosis or health problems that interested me. I could never begin to tell you the vital signs on the monitor when we rushed into the patient's room, or what medications were running and at what rate, or the name of the doctors who rushed into the room with the precipitous basin. There were so many things about that day and that patent that I will never forget. Her families' face is forever inscribed in my mind, surprisingly each has a smile. I will never forget her name or the ten week old little boy to who she gave birth. She had, within one hour's time, changed my life forever.

It was later that night when I was sitting at home staring at the television, still in shock, that I realized no matter how much the events of the day had affected me, they had also showed me I had chosen the career that was meant for me. She and her family were a few of the most amazing people I had ever been blessed enough to meet, much less provide care. I was changed that day, both as a nurse and a person, and I hope to carry and share that memory for the rest of my career. I think of her and her family often and I find I still smile each time.

Kimberly Theriot, BSN, RN

A Memorable Couple

An incident happened during my third semester clinical rotation which has moved me so much that I decided nursing is my true calling. It is for this profession that I have waited for so long in my life to start. A man in his fifties in the Intensive Care Unit diagnosed with liver cancer and his wife at the bedside holding his hands and weeping – a scene I think that I can never forget. His cancer was detected at the last stage, and he was drawing near to his final days. He couldn't speak but could understand everything he heard. His wife kept on talking to him in Spanish. She talked to me about their story – how much they loved each other, the initial struggle when they came to the United States and raising their kids, etc. I spent considerable longer time that day with them talking to the wife. I encouraged her to talk more about her feelings. Surprisingly she went back in to the past describing about their journey from Mexico to the United States, her initial struggle in learning English, and the small jobs that she did in the beginning. She was talking in such a manner that she included her husband also in the conversation, and I noticed that the patient was listening and tears coming out of his eyes. I went back to the room as I was about to leave for the day. My patient's wife said that she felt more courageous and ready to accept the fact that he would die any moment after talking with me. It was a defining moment in my nursing school days that I felt a sort of fulfillment inside my heart. Her kind words gave me even greater motivation to continue nursing and make meaningful effects on the lives of my patients and their families.

Antony Thomas, BSN, RN

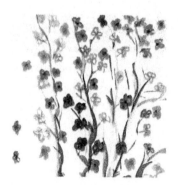

My First Code Blue

The moment I knew nursing was it for me was during my first ever code blue which happened during my first semester. It wasn't my patient, but she was an elderly woman who had seized and then coded. At first I was extremely hesitant on entering the room. But once I had that push from my clinical instructor, which I am very thankful for, I was really able to see what was being done and all the fast paced attempts that were going on in efforts to save the patient. Personally, this being my first ever actual Code Blue, I froze on the spot! Even though my adrenaline was pumping, I could not believe it was really happening! Afterward, I felt like I didn't provide my full potential because I believe I did not contribute to anything

Everything seemed to have gone a million miles an hour. The code cart arrived in the room; a rush of people followed not too long after which included a team consisting of people such as a doctor, respiratory therapist, nurses, the code team, and I'm sure there were more. During the entire event there were thought processes being discussed, history of the patient was being given, report of medications given, and anything else that could help determine the next steps that should be involved. Meanwhile the patient was laying there unresponsive to what was going on around her. During the entire situation while I was trying to figure out what was exactly happening, I was shocked at how much the people involved managed to remember throughout the entire stressful event. Ultimately the decision was made to intubate her. It was crazy; the intense emotional roller coaster that the nurses had gone through at that moment. But at the end they got her back just fine. Seeing how their facial expressions of accomplishment made me feel like, "This is it. I want to become a nurse." Even though it is an intense and emotional experience, it is also a very rewarding experience knowing that you make such a difference in someone's life. You just have to have your head in the right place for the benefit of the patient.

Ashley Thomas, BSN, RN

Patient Reflection

It was second semester of nursing school and my first day in the Neonatal Intensive Care Unit (NICU). I was assigned to a 37-week premature newborn baby girl whom I learned was the only survivor of triplets after being resuscitated. The doctors thought her chances of surviving and having no cerebral damage was very slim. Not to mention, her mother was also in the Intensive Care Unit (ICU) and had a 50% chance of surviving. Mother and daughter were both fighting for their lives. Throughout this ordeal, the father lost all color in him and was clinging to the only faith he had left. Throughout the midst of monitoring my patient, the NICU nurse called me in an isolated room along with a fellow student. I was shocked when I entered the room because lying there were two beautiful babies with dark red lips, dressed in white dresses. They were lifeless. It broke my heart when I found out they were my patient's sisters. We took their footprints and made plaster casts out of them, cut portions of their hair, took their pictures and created a beautiful memory box for the family. We swaddled the babies prior to showing them to the family. It was the hardest thing to see, but knowing I was able to make something for the family that they'll be able to treasure forever brought me comfort. A month later, I learned that the mother and baby both survived with no further complications. The news brought tears to my eyes. Their courage and will to live motivated and remained me of why I chose the nursing profession.

Christela Turner, BSN, RN

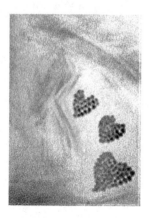

Unforeseeable Forces

When I started nursing school, there was no doubt where I would work. "Pediatric Oncology" I would say when people and friends would inquire where I wanted to work. The reaction was always the same, one of incredible hurt, then shock. "Why on Earth would you want to work there, it is so sad. I could never do that." The thing is I have never seen it as a sad place. In fact, despite my reputation for being an almost ridiculously emotional person, I have only cried once, and the situation is not what I expected.

My third day on a pediatric oncology floor proved to be my answer to the standard, "Why do you want to work there?" question. The answer had evaded me for my whole four years of school despite my eagerness to be with those children. In three short days, among my rounds of vital signs and dinner tray delivery I had seen so much living among the poor prognosis. I watched as a young child of nine had turned to her mother and matter-of-factly stated that she would not be returning home. She seemed sad that she would not see her home again, seemingly nonchalant about the fact that her short life would soon be over. I walked in and out of the dimly lit rooms, the air thick with an emotion that I would not wish on anyone. An occasional smile and greeting was offered to the patient and family, yet I didn't feel like I was making a difference in the encounters with these brave patients. I realized that the difference I wanted to make was not a promise of a cure, or to take their pain away, simply I wanted them to smile. That is why I became a nurse. If I could make their time in the hospital better, even if for one moment, it would all be worth it and the question I have always been asked would be answered.

The next day on the floor, I walked into a fourteen year old girl's room. Just a week before, I had watched her being wheeled in shortly after biopsy surgery. Her parents followed the gurney, eyes red and swollen, shoulders hunched as not to be disturbed. They knew the diagnosis, the girl did not. This day, she was sitting up in bed, chemotherapy medication hanging from a pole beside her. She had not lost her hair, something that as teenagers we take for granted. She still looked sad; her life had been changed forever. I started wrapping the blood pressure cuff around her upper arm, making small talk as I went. I wanted so bad to know how this little girl had been before. I wondered if she laughed and played with her friends, experienced life as it should be. Not here in this hospital. I offered to paint her toenails, something I had heard made a young patient feel better. She kindly declined and looked back down in her lap. I decided to tell her a joke. Simple enough. If nothing else, the mother who was always so faithfully by her side would smile. I didn't ask, just started. When I asked the question portion, she looked up at me in shock. Why was I telling her a joke in the hospital? Was this allowed? The environment was sterile and cold, could humor find a place here? When I perfectly delivered my punch line, nothing less than a miracle (to me at least) occurred. Unrestricted, bellyaching, smile from ear to ear and a laugh that was music to my heart. The poor girl was red and holding her tummy, hysterical and I knew at that moment why I was there.

Kathryn [Lawson] Vaello, BNS, RN

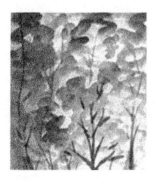

An Uncooperative Patient

I was told that the patient I was about to speak with was violent, uncooperative, and unpleasant. The staff members were not too fond of the young man. I watched him sitting quietly, scribbling away in a journal. He scanned the room with a suspicious eye but failed to make eye contact when I approached him. I asked him how his day was coming along. His responses were mostly one word answers, short and to the point. I pulled up a chair and asked him about his writing. At first he was a bit hesitant to speak with me, but his face lit up when he started telling me of his journal, stories, and his aspiration to write a novel. Showing an interest in his interests made him feel at ease, and he opened up about his condition and his family life. The family he described was very dysfunctional, abusive, and unsupportive. He had many vulnerabilities and had been incredibly hurt throughout his lifetime. His situation was complex and misunderstood by those around him. He told me how nurses gave him medications but never spoke with him, and that they did not seem to care. His concerns were often dismissed. He felt alone and upset. I spent some time speaking with him, allowing the conversation to flow openly but ultimately returning to the matter of his care and his end goals. He told me in the most sincere tone, "You're a very good listener," and smiled a warm smile. His behavior changed drastically that day, and the staff even commented on it. I felt happy that I could affect a patient in a positive way just by genuine communication. I knew at that moment that I was exactly where I needed to be.

Angelica Valle, BSN, RN

A Homeless Patient

Ralph* was a malnourished, homeless man. He weighed less than one-hundred pounds on admission. At the beginning, I remember how Ralph would curse something evil every time someone would bother him to take vital signs, ask questions, etc. His reaction was especially agitated and aggressive during more invasive procedures (e.g. during tube and IV placement). Ralph was so disagreeable at one time that he flung stool from his colostomy bag at hospital staff. Food was a comfort for Ralph, though. After all, he was hungry! He would eat three trays of food at each meal. Consequently, he was emptying his colostomy bag at least three times every eight hours. After several weeks of eating ample amounts of food he gained over twenty pounds. Ralph was most happy when he was fed, and slowly the poop-slinging and cursing ceased. He became more sociable and friendly as time went along. I was amazed to watch this man struggle with loneliness, hunger, and lack of shelter. As Ralph's basic needs were fulfilled he became more receptive to communicating with others and following his treatment regimen. Unfortunately, not one person came to visit Ralph during his hospital stay. Nursing staff, along with the social worker and chaplain, helped prepare Ralph to manage his health beyond discharge and build connections with shelters in the community to help him during difficult times. Ralph is a premier example of why I got into nursing. He is someone who really had no one to call upon for help or even a hug. To show apathy toward the lame and homeless renders us inhuman. Ralph reminded me that someone cares, no matter how bad things get in our lives. Sometimes, that someone is a nurse!

Russell VanBremen, BSN,

*The patient's name was changed to protect patient confidentially.

A Busy Day

As a student, it wasn't until the last semester, that I actually started feeling like a real nurse. The floor I was working on was real busy, and I was assigned to four patients. Time management was out the window. Starting the shift in the morning and completing the assessments was not easy. Upon arriving three call lights were going off. Two patients needed pain medication, and one patient needed wound care as soon as possible. Unfortunately, these were tasks that could not be delegated to a tech. That day I learned why our instructors had taught us how to do quick assessments. Up until that day, as students, we were able perform thorough assessments. So I grabbed the pain medications, and as I administered the pain medications, I did my assessment on both patients. Then I went and grabbed my supplies for wound care and again did my quick assessment. Just when I thought I could breath, eight o'clock medications were due. So I pulled out my medications that were now due only to realize that the blood sugars for my patients had not been taken. It turns out that our floor was short a tech! The day continued to be this busy throughout the entire day. Boy, was I overwhelmed. I felt like I could not please my patients because I was stretched so thin. I honestly felt inadequate as a nurse. I was barely satisfying my patients, and I was barely keeping my nursing tasks on schedule. However, in the mist of this busy day, I was able to bond with a patient of mine. This patient was a diabetic, and he was admitted to the hospital for complications from his diabetes. From the chart, this patient is what you call an uncompliant diabetic, but after speaking with this patient, I learned he was a very loving father and deeply wanted to help his children go far and become successful in life. It was very touching. I was able to give patient teaching about his diabetes. What was different about this time from the hundred times he had heard it since his diagnosis was that he let me know what was important to him, his children. After my teaching, he thanked me and was almost in tears. He stated, he had never seen it from that perspective before. I can't predict in the future he would be more compliant, but I know that day he realized in order to help his children; he needed to start with himself, which is an accomplishment. I was able to walk off the floor with a smile because that's exactly the reason why I joined nursing.

Raquel Villasenor, BSN, RN

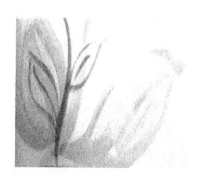

Intensive Care Unit Mother

I don't know what I would do if my child ended up in the Intensive Care Unit (ICU). The way I view things now, I do not want one of my babies hooked up to machines for an extended period of time. As a nurse, my job is to care for this patient without judgment and without opinion about the family's decisions. I was touched not by a patient I encountered, but her mother. This patient was fairly young and had been in a horrible car accident a couple months before, leaving her unresponsive to everything except pain. This patient was on a ventilator and did not take any breaths on her own, requiring every biological need to be met by either a machine or a nurse. My first thoughts were: "Why extend the sufferings of this poor child? When does being sustained by medical interventions surpass the will to die?" Then I met her mother. Such a beautiful and hopeful woman came to the patient's bedside. She talked to her daughter and told her she was there with a comforting voice. She washed each of her hands, exfoliating off the dead tissue and applying lotion, carefully massaging it on her hands. From this mother I learned one huge valuable lesion: Hope. Where are we without it? Who are we as nurses that stand back and judge these prolonging life measures? Honestly, after seeing that mom, I had to rethink about what I would do if I were in the same situation.

Amanda Wholly, BSN, RN

A Very Bad or Bored Patient

I was receiving my hand off report from the RN coming off her night shift. During the report we were interrupted by one of the alarms on the mechanical ventilator because the patient had disconnected the ventilator from his trachea collar. The night RN, who was obviously very tired and frustrated from her long shift, went into the room and stated, "He's being a very bad boy, you should give him his benzo early so you can have a peaceful shift. He's been a nightmare." She stated it so plainly as if the patient was not even in the room. She reconnected the ventilator and we left the room to continue with the hand off report. A few moments later we were interrupted again by the alarm. The night nurse entered the room and as she was connecting the ventilator for the second time said to the patient, "If you don't stop being such a bad boy, I'm going to restrain you." Before we even left the room the patient had disconnected his ventilator yet again. The night RN restrained both of the patient's hands to the bed and said, "Happy now?" When we walked out of the room the RN said, "You should give him his benzo now so he'll sleep for the next few hours till his mom gets here and you can actually get some work done." I told the RN that he was probably just bored because he's 10 years old and the only thing to keep him occupied was a 30 minute episode of Veggie Tales playing on repeat in his room. I walked into the room and let the patient pick out a new movie to watch and changed it for him.

Meanwhile the charge nurse came in with a toy and sat with the patient and played with him for the next hour and he did not pull out his ventilator again. She even had him smiling a little. I realized then how thankful I was that I chose to be a nurse. I wanted to be in a profession to help people. I had no idea that most help was just from the care and not even involving medical treatment. The hospital is not a place that people are excited to be, but knowing that I aided in making that stay a little brighter just by listening instead of cutting someone short could make all the difference in a person's stay. I know that the night nurse is probably a very good nurse and all good people can have a bad day. But I chose nursing so I could make a difference, and I hope to do that every day I step into the hospital because you never know what difference you can make in a person's life with a simple smile.

Kristy Zorn, BSN, RN

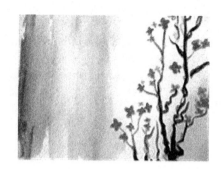

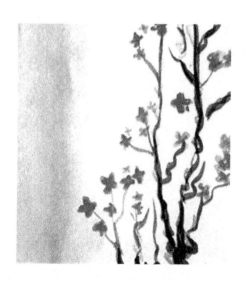

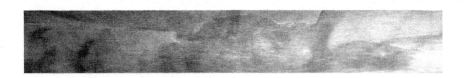

A Challenge

After reading this book, I'm sure you have noticed that the one thing the students learned was that nursing is more than just pushing medications. Nursing really is about caring. They also noted that the one complaint patients mentioned the most was that nurses did not have time to spend or talk with them.

My challenge to all nurses is this. Remember the reasons you became a nurse. Even though there are times when you are extremely busy, spend some time talking with your patients, even if is only five minutes. Listen to your patients. Don't be one of the nurses that patients tell students, "My nurse doesn't have time to talk with me or answer my questions."

Beverly Wheeler

CPSIA information can be obtained at www.ICGtesting.com
Printed in the USA
BVOW08*0137110516

447627BV00001B/2/P